Prognosis for a Septuagenarian/Octogenarian

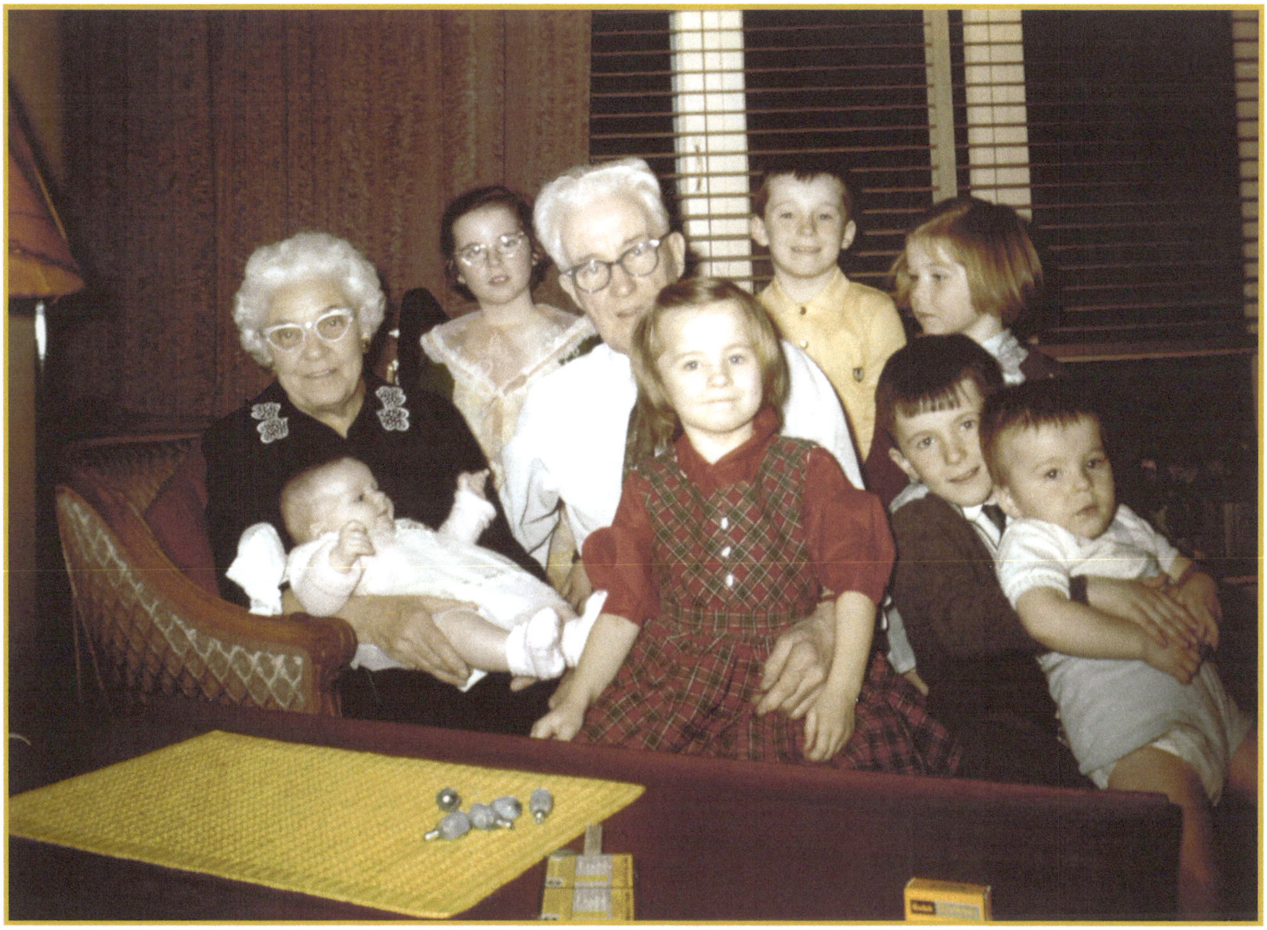

*The Author's parents, **Michael Tansey** & **Charlotte Hunter**
with 7 of their 15 grandchildren*

Standing: *Cathy Tansey, Timothy Summers, Patricia Tansey,*

Seated: *Charlotte Summers (on Grandma's knee),
Elizabeth Summers (on Grandpa's knee), Nicholas Summers
with Patrick Summers (on his knee)*

*This book is dedicated to my late sister, Charlotte Hunter Tansey,
for her wisdom and sincerity in dealing with students,
her staff and the public in her 64 years in the
Education Field in Montreal, Quebec, Canada.*

Copyright © CarTan 2013

ISBN 978-0-9696738-3-5

All rights reserved

No part of this book may be reproduced in any form, by photostat, microfilm, xerography, or any other means, or incorporated into any information retrieval system, electronic or mechanical, without the written permission of the copyright owner.

Publisher: CarTan, Montreal, Canada

Graphic Design and Production: Jacqueline Dawson

Photography: Photos from the Tansey and Hunter Family Archives

Front Cover Photo: Cynthia Soares

Michael & Charlotte
(Lot, Lottie)

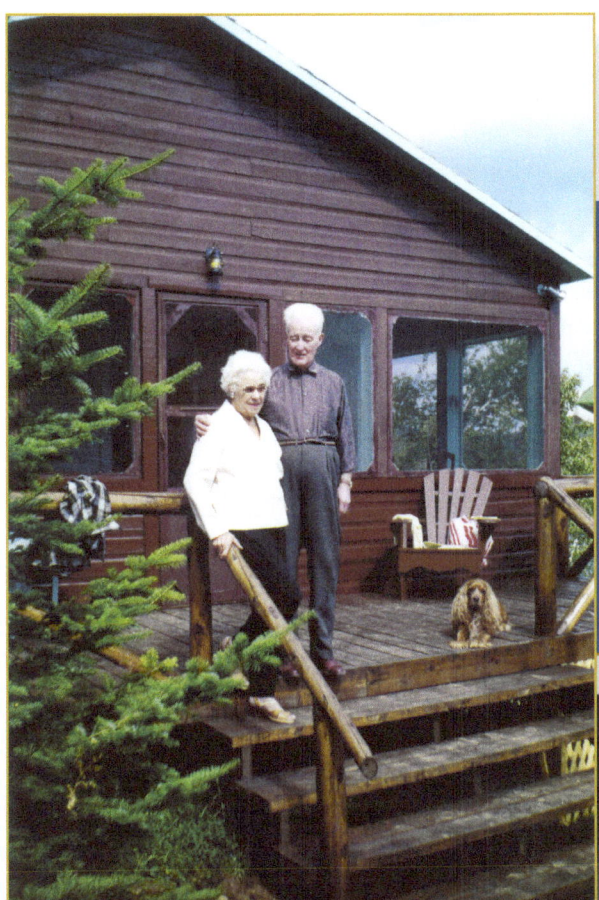

At the country house in The Laurentians

With the author, Carol Tansey, on board the Queen Elizabeth

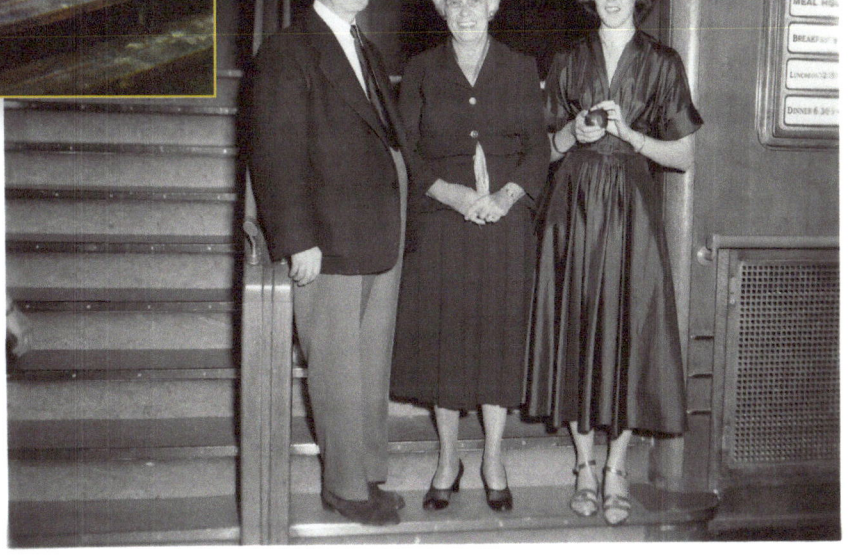

*This book contains many pictures of Seniors because
I am building credibility with the reader for my interest and
concern for Seniors. My Mother was a few weeks short of
40 years old when I was born, and my Father was a few weeks
short of 46. So, you will understand that I have lived with and
loved older folks all my life. And now that I am one of them
I believe that I understand them, too.*

CONTENTS

Family & Ancestor Pictures
.... *i. iii, 11-13, 16, 51-61*

Contents .... *v*

Introduction *1*

Poems—Written In 2004 .... *5*

Obviously Not My Time To Go *7*

*And They Wonder Why Seniors
Think Of Suicide* *8*

Hunger *14*

Nutrition and Cooking *17*

More Poetry *20*

Where I Ended Up *21*

Drugs & Things *22*

Gluten Free Diet *24*

*The Reason Why I Am Asking
For A Change Of Residence* *29*

Nursing Care *33*

PABS *35*

Religion *36*

Auxiliary *36*

Medical Care *36*

Therapy *36*

Foot Care *36*

Hair Salon *36*

Nutrition *36*

IDT *37*

Residents' Committee *38*

Coordinators *38*

Ombudsperson *38*

Laundry *39*

Maintenance & Cleaning *40*

Teeth *41*

Glasses *41*

Walking *42*

Computer *43*

Itchy Skin & Bloody Nose *44*

A Sad Moment *44*

Room Safety *44*

Outside Physicians' Appointments *45*

Entertainment *45*

Sum Up *46*

*My Ancestors &
The Montreal Community* *48*

Recommendations *62*

About the Author *65*

Introduction

"*She will not recover. As you see her now, she will be until she dies.*"

This prognosis was given to my sister when I was discharged from hospital in July 2007, after having had seven strokes in six months—from February to July.

Don't be so quick to write me off! Six years later I am still here!

I am well aware that I could have another stroke and die tomorrow or be bedridden for several years. I prefer to take a lighter, more hopeful approach to life, and while I will attempt to bring you some humorous things that happen in a nursing home setting, I am also absolutely serious about things that could make life more pleasant for the elderly and the sick.

I have written two Gluten-Free cookbooks since I have been in the second long-term care center, and this book, now in progress, about my six years as an in-house paying guest of the Quebec Medicare System.

On the lighter side, today there was a new PAB (Préposée aux bénéficiaire) working on our floor, but she didn't come near me until the day was nearly over. When questioned about it, she said they had told her that I didn't like new faces! Truth is that there are far too many new faces—but I don't dislike every new face on sight!

Six years ago, in early February, I was found on the floor in the apartment I was sharing with my sister, who was in hospital at the time. I had gotten up, gone to the bathroom, taken the lock off the front door for the CLSC worker (from the Local Health Care Center), who was coming later, and started back to bed (only I didn't make it), so was found on the floor. I regained consciousness in the ambulance about four hours later.

Now I want to take you through the last six years and tell you what life is like in hospital and in two long-term care facilities in Montreal, Canada, and how I came to receive Potty Training at 81 and an Introduction to Pole Dancing at 82.

In February 2007 I became a prisoner of the diaper—yet it beats a catheter or a wet bed. Some time ago I thought "If we can train a two year old, we can train an octogenarian," and I was ready to step out and move into pull-ups—at least in the daytime hours.

I will spare you the details—enough to say that progress is being made, with lots of kind help. One must be positive, and insist on action with the cooperation of management. Workers are usually helpful, though not always. You must study yourself—When do you need the help?—and ask for it seriously.

When we achieve small successes we are so happy, and sometimes the cheering section is with us. It is rather odd how we must reduce our aims to suit the workings of the institution. The resident seems often to be the last one considered, even when we think we have made a firm arrangement with a staff person. Sometimes I wonder if staff know or care how their actions affect the residents?

This might be an appropriate time to ask—does management ever inform staff about residents who have had strokes, and let them know that therefore their emotions are very much on or close to surface level? We laugh easily, we cry easily, we are upset easily, and we are frustrated easily. It might be useful if residents were cut a little slack on this point.

However, I do appreciate the fact that the staff, in the two institutions in which my sister and I have made our home for the last few years (until my sister's death in August 2010) have been kind to us. But really, does it need to take three PABs to push a juice cart at 1:30 pm? That is what just passed my door, and yet sometimes it is difficult to get changed!

In July 2007, I was admitted to the first long-term care facility, which was a private institution, while waiting for a government facility. To achieve admittance to the government facility a person must submit their last six months bank statements, be medically certified as to the number of hours of nursing care per week required, and then wait for a space. The government then fixes the monthly rent and board (which is usually less than private), and leaves you with a very small allowance. In my case the allowance is currently $297.41 per month.

With this allowance you must pay for any other needs or wants, such as hair care, foot care, dental care, clothing purchases, telephone, cable TV, internet, kleenex, deodorant, polident and cosmetics. *(The Government does give some grants for a percentage of dentures, glasses, orthopaedic shoes and cataract surgery for low income residents.)*

And, if you want to have a cup of tea or ice cream in the Tuck Shop—that costs money too. Or, if you have to visit a relative in hospital who is in grave condition, and you must use the medi-car (as I did several times because I am in a wheelchair) the cost is by the mile and by the hour. The Government calls this a social call and the resident must pay for it. How can you survive? Do you beg, borrow or steal?

On exit from the facility, a family must remove all of a person's effects within 24-48 hours. There is always somebody else waiting.

This doesn't give one a very hopeful end-of-life period. When you are old and sick and poor, it is very hard to find joy in your life.

Suddenly you are unimportant, worthless, not taken seriously, talked down to, not believed, and certainly not encouraged to do anything to help yourself. Dignity and respect are gone. Your dignity flies out the door if you have forgotten to close the window when you are sitting on the commode as the door flies open. I have had unexpected visits from the higher to the lower staff. I find it unsettling and off-putting. Do parents not teach children manners any more? A door which is usually open is closed—it is closed for a reason. The polite thing to do would be to knock and wait for a reply. Probably the men are just amused by this when they come upon me. Just because you need the help of a nursing home does not mean it is open season for all.

As for the workers—some are very kind and dedicated, some are fairly kind, but do only what they think is their duty and not a bit more, and then there are those who seem to come for the paycheque alone.

It is a hopeless situation I find myself in. There are so many things that I want to do, but I am physically unable to do them. I find it hard to ask for help, when for years I have been able to do so many things for myself. And other people are busy doing their own thing.

So you give up trying, and withdraw more and more into yourself. But when someone can give you a few minutes you are so grateful. Were we so miserable with our generosity of time when we were able-bodied?

I can remember as a young teenager visiting my grandmother often—going shopping with her, accompanying her to the bank, going with her to the cemetery. Was I different? Is that why I expect more from the able-bodied now? What happened to volunteerism? What happened to people just enjoying each other?

And yet, as I ask these questions I realize how lucky I am. Two of my nieces, Cathy and Patricia, visited me last evening. Cathy took me out for a drive last week. Jacqui, another niece, called from Florida, to tell me she was sending me a new TV for Christmas, and another niece from Newfoundland, Elizabeth, called to say that she was putting me on the Internet at Christmas time.

I guess I am just greedy and oh so lucky, but there are another 133 residents in this same institution (34 of them on this floor alone)—some have very faithful families—some do not!

POEMS
Written in 2004, many feelings the same in 2013

Health Care Ststem in Montreal

She lies in her bed
No doctor will come near
She says she's not well
But no one will hear.

She has some good friends
But family are scarce
Fifteen nephews and nieces
And visits are rare
Snail mail and email exist
But few seem to care.

Siblings are all very poorly
But fingers do dial
So empathy abounds
And siblings do care.

Family Medicine and CLSCs
Operate apart from the rest
Where efficiency and compassion
Do exist—but are rare.

ERs are slow—hot and variable
Some are great—some are degrading
Diagnoses are slow
2-4 months is the norm
It's not fast for treatment
To get back in form.

Some doctors in hospital excel
One surgeon in expertise
And communication did well
Some doctors are kind
While others are crude
Some humiliate
While others light up a room
With hope and with cheer.

Some nurses dominate
While others are professional
Helpful and kind
Some night nurses rule
By intimidation and fear
Some day nurses proudly announce
"We don't wash feet here."

Technicians do well
Orderlies excel
Pastoral Services have great personnel
In short a mixed bag does prevail.

POEMS CONTINUED

MY SPUNK IS SPENT

My spunk is spent

My manners are gone

I burp like a teenage boy

The hair needs a trim

The toenails too

The legs get weaker

The teeth want attention

The skin gets patchy and red

The lines under the eyes get deeper and blacker

The balance is shot, the dizziness looms

Dignity, elegance, and beauty are gone

And where are courage and self confidence?

And coping skills?

We now are dependent on pills

Some days are bad, some days not so

But we wake every day with trepidation and woe

This is the time when inner beauty must shine

And not from so many x-rays that we glow!

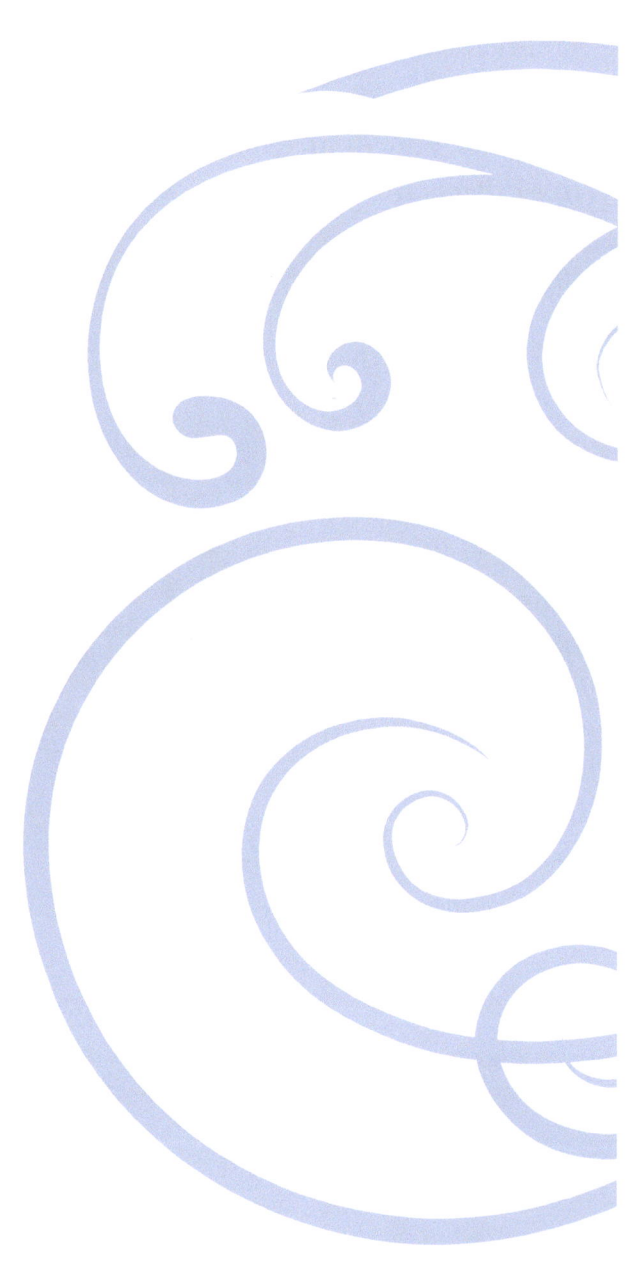

Obviously Not My Time To Go

I guess it was not my time to go, no matter what the hospital and the government had decided. Between them they decided I was only worthy of being kept clean and fed—but not of being given any hope or therapy. So I fooled them!

After a year and a half of waiting to die, and wishing I was dead, I decided to try to write my name. A friend suggested it would be good to be able to sign a cheque! I had not been able to do anything for myself. It would be a good thing to be able to do, in case I won the lotto!

A nurse brought me in a copybook that her child had not used in school, and a pen. And I started, first with the left hand, then the right (which was my normal writing hand), then both hands. After weeks and many pages—I could write my name. Then I started on the alphabet, in capitals, lower case letters, numbers, sentences, paragraphs. So I feel I can write now—it is painful and slow—but it is possible.

Another nurse hid a wheelchair near me so that I could learn to drive it. The one I had was too cumbersome, I could not manage it. We practised with it many days and I was doing well with it, until it was found in my cupboard one day, and taken from me. About the same time my own wheelchair was adjusted, and that stopped my writing. Somehow they made the chair's arms impossible for my arms to move any more. I cried so much—it just seemed that I was being denied anything I had worked so hard to achieve. I wanted to die so badly.

But it still wasn't my time!

About that time, we were moved from the private institution to the government administered one, and things improved a little, though there is still room for improvement. We were warned that life would be more difficult here, which was not true.

And They Wonder Why Seniors Think of Suicide

Let me tell you why. When I was released from hospital in July 2007 to a long-term care center, after being in hospital for 6 months and having suffered 7 strokes, the prognosis my sister received for me was:

"SHE WILL NOT RECOVER. AS YOU SEE HER NOW, SHE WILL BE UNTIL SHE DIES."

I was refused therapy from that day on. I do receive some now in the second long-term center—they call it Maintenance Therapy.

Having received no hope from the Government or the Management of the Center, and having Medicare charging me most of my pension for room and board, life is not great, and I do get depressed!

15 times I have stopped eating and drinking. I simply did not want to live any more. One time a nurse said to me, "If you wanted to eat—what would you like?" I thought for a minute, and then thinking she will never be able to find it at 10 o'clock at night in a nursing home, I asked for cheesecake. The joke was on me. She found it. She stood there and fed it to me—as I was shaking too much to cope. And I realised that she had won that round. She then gave me a very short speech about how we had to fight this on a full stomach—not an empty one.

Another nurse in the first center had advised me that I must learn to appreciate what I can do and not dwell on what I cannot.

About one year after I was discharged from hospital, my brain came back. In the last five years I have involved myself in the following projects:

1. *I taught myself to write again.*
2. *I relearned the computer.*
3. *I have had major teeth repairs.*
4. *I consulted a gastroenterologist for Gluten Sensitivity Disease*

5. *I was featured in the Canadian Celiac Association Spring Newsletter, the Quebec Celiac News and the Suburban.*
6. *I have written and published two Gluten Free cookbooks.*
7. *I have taken back the management of my affairs.*
8. *I have become Executor and Beneficiary of my sister's Estate.*
9. *I started Potty Training at 81 years of age.*
10. *I had an Introduction to Pole Dancing at 82 years.*
11. *I am presently working on this book called Prognosis for a Septuagenarian/Octogenarian which covers my 6 years as a paying guest—in-house—with the Quebec Medicare System*
12. *I am considering eye surgery for cataracts.*
13. *I am struggling very hard to walk again.*
14. *I have consulted a Surgeon in Podiatry.*

In August 2010 I had to watch my sister die of complications from Diabetes. She lost most of her sight, her heart and kidneys gave trouble—in short all her systems just gave up. She was in terrible pain and asked us to help her. She had wanted so much to live.

I did consult Medical and Religious Advisers as well as friends and relatives. The consensus of opinion seemed to be that I should make it as easy as possible for her—but it still hurt me unbelievably.

And so I learned that life is very precious and that I should appreciate what I can do and not dwell on what I cannot.

I feel people could be kinder to each other.

I think Therapy should be available to the elderly who want it.

I believe government should charge seniors as they charge for children in daycare and let them have hope and a little more cash.

A great part of the reason for suicide is lack of hope—but I do not condone Suicide. You can get much satisfaction from your achievements—if you have hope.

We must listen to friends and relatives when they feel terribly frustrated due to the hopeless situation that they feel they are in.

There is always a solution. A special word to all, and especially to health care workers —**LISTEN**.

Please believe me—I have been there.

Read further in this book, in the chapter on Gluten Free Diet for Gluten Sensitivity Disease, and you will learn about the difficulty that I have had with getting credibility and diet to achieve comfort with this problem.

One day about a year ago I came close to ending it all when I was served a lunch of a large white round bun, which was then replaced by a long white bun, which was replaced by a brown bread sandwich—as if changing the shape or color could turn the ingredients into becoming gluten-free! I have been here for five years and the message is still not clear to the kitchen that I must not have wheat flour! Continual ingesting, when there is a need to be gluten free, can lead to terrible pain, diarrhea and possibly even Colon Cancer (which I have already suffered through, and had surgery for, once).

My niece, who came to see me that night, kept asking "Why didn't anyone listen to Carol? She has studied Nutrition and she knows exactly what she can eat and what she can't."

I was very frustrated and felt that the kitchen would never realize the importance of the situation, and management would never make sure that they did.

Within seconds, I had changed my mind and thought 'you better be very sure of what you are doing'. And I am pleased to be still alive.

On looking back, it seems pretty silly to lose my life because of two white buns and two pieces of brown bread!

My word to all — **LISTEN** — to friends and relatives and to those in your care.

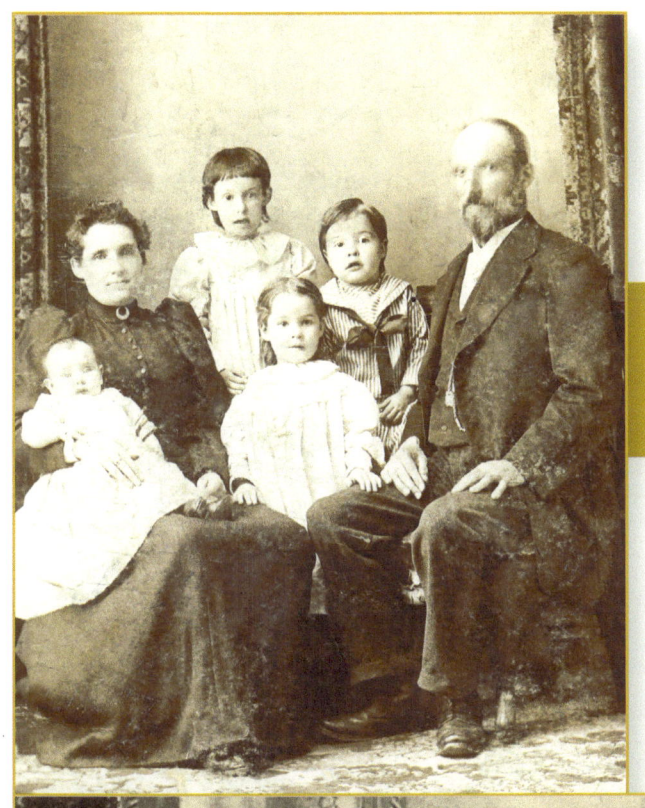

Mother's Side of the Family

Seated: **Grandma Hunter** with **Baby Jessie**, **Grandpa Hunter**, circa 1895

Standing (back to front): **Elizabeth, James & Charlotte** (the author's mother)

> And then there are our ancestors on both sides of the family...

Father's Side of the Family

Grandpa & Grandma Tansey with their children, circa 1899

Seated: **Margaret, Mamie, Rosemary**

Standing: **Tom, Sara, Michael** (the author's father)

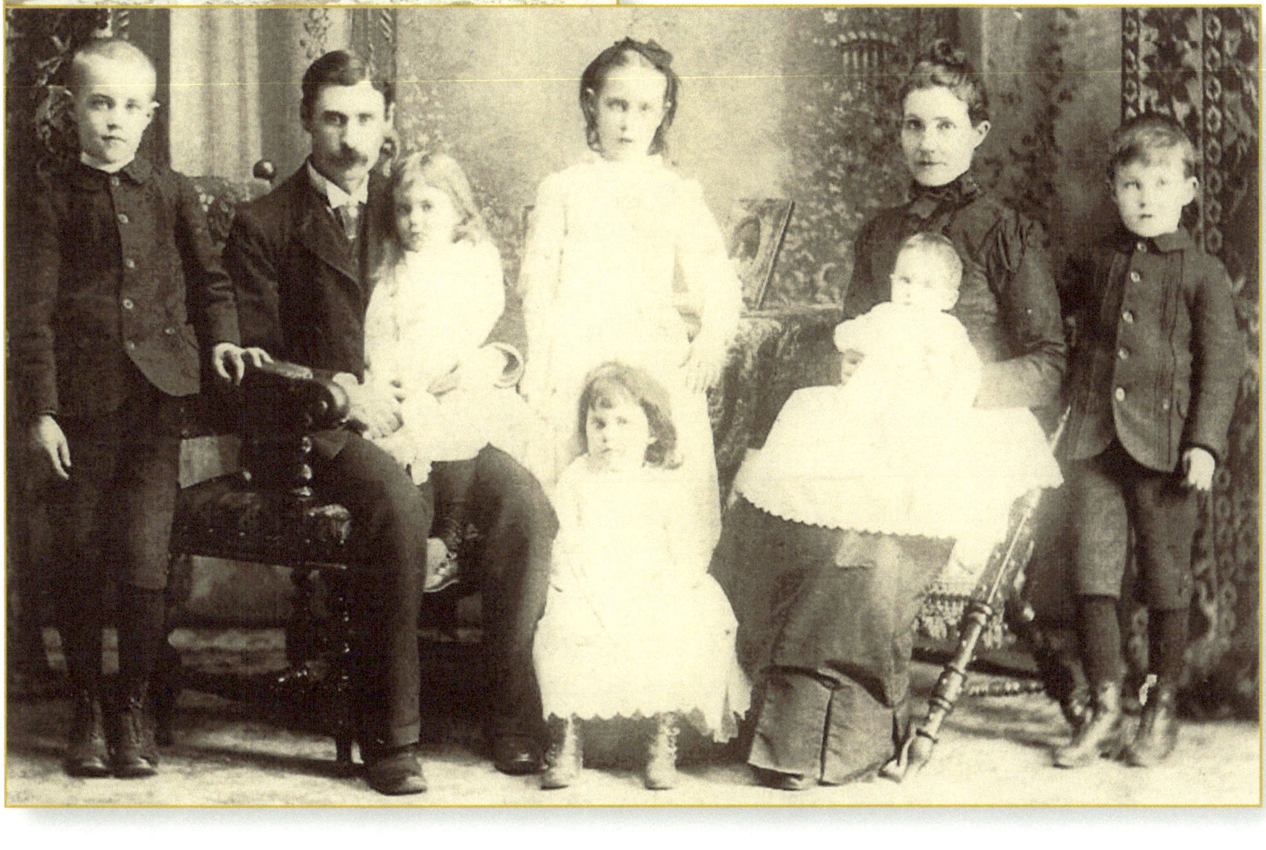

The Five Children of Michael & Lot

Facing page, as young adults circa 1947: (clockwise from top left) **Charlotte, Barbara, Peter, Mary & Carol**

Since we have all lived to reach beyond 80 we do claim to know a little about Octogenarians.

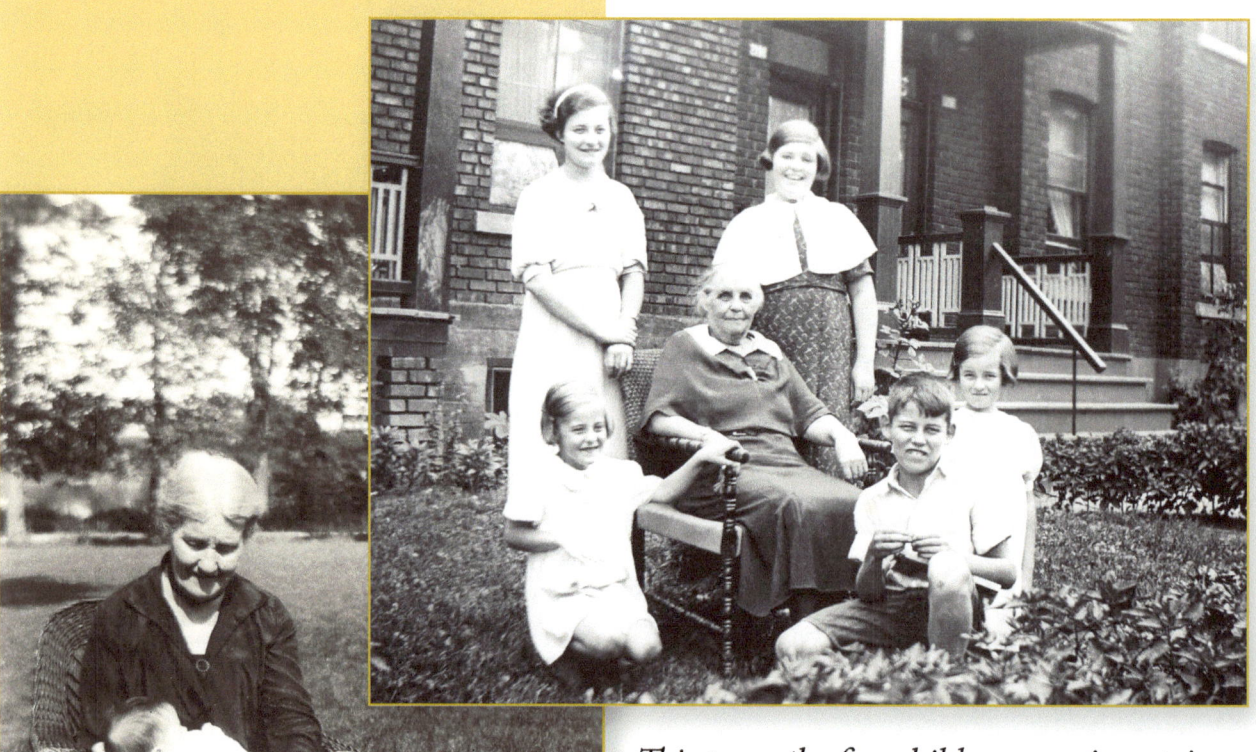

This page, the five children growing up in The Depression with their grandmothers.

Above: **Grandma Hunter** *with (clockwise from top left)* **Charlotte, Barbara, Mary, Peter & Carol,** *circa 1934.*

Left: **Grandma Tansey** *with (clockwise from bottom right)* **Charlotte, Peter, Barbara & Baby Mary,** *circa 1925. (Carol has not yet arrived.)*

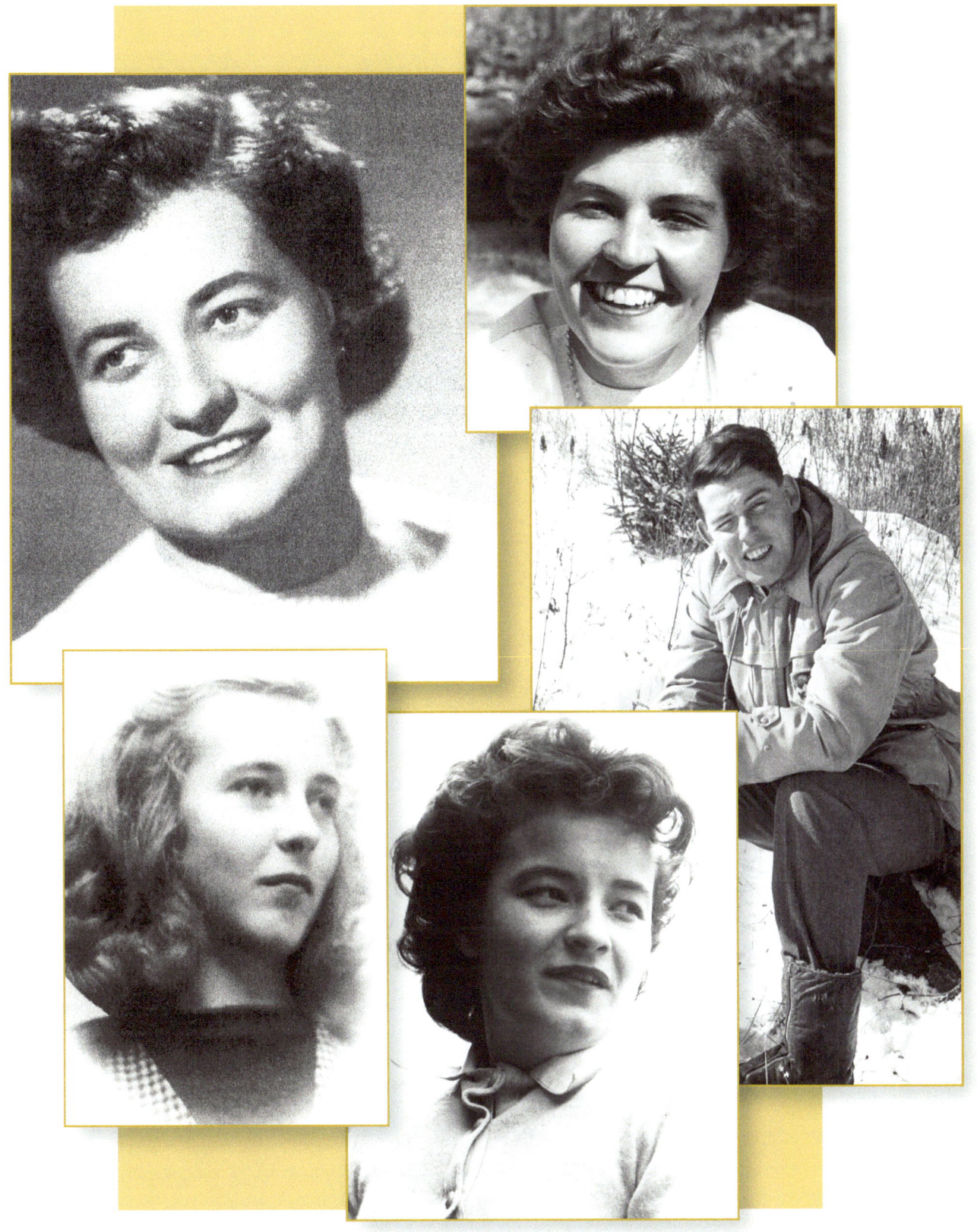

Hunger

1929 *DEPRESSION YEAR—I was born.*

And yet, I never knew HUNGER—until now. Now, when I am old and ill and in a nursing home, the attitude towards the elderly seems to be 'lie in your bed and die, take your pills and don't make trouble'.

We were five children, my father out of work, my mother beside herself trying to feed and care for us all, my father walking miles to get bread for five cents a loaf, instead of ten cents, my two older sisters running behind coal trucks, picking up pieces of coal to warm us. And yet, I never remember HUNGER. Somehow my mother got a bone from the butcher, a few potatoes, a few carrots and onions, and with dumplings she made a big pot of soup. And with the bread we were fed. Sometimes my mother would cut the hair of the girls next door (there were five of them) and their father would give us a bag of tomatoes from his garden. The neighbour upstairs would give us some wood—when she had some. Neighbours were more kind to each other in that era.

I tell you these things so that you will understand that even though we did suffer in The DEPRESSION, I did not know HUNGER until I had several strokes and needed to be in a long-term care facility.

All five children did grow up and reach university-level education with many degrees, diplomas, honours, etc.—but all with bad teeth because of poor nutrition in the Depression years.

While in hospital during the months of suffering the strokes, I was prepared several times for sending to a Rehab center, but each time I had another stroke. The government likes you to show improvement quickly and if you don't within a prescribed time you are declared hopeless and long-term. They should not have given up on me so quickly.

Once I was declared hopeless, I received no Speech Therapy, no Mental Therapy, no Physiotherapy, no Therapy of any kind—

zilch. I was on my own. My job was to die. Only I didn't! After waiting a year and a half to die, I decided somebody should be in charge of me—so it might as well be me.

But to get back to HUNGER, which was the purpose of this chapter—many nights I have gone to bed hungry. The staff would tell me just to ask for something. I find it hard to beg for food.

However, to beg for food was quite an effort. First I met with the IDT group (an Inter Disciplinary Team of about seven members), then to a meeting called by the Executive Director (again about seven members—mostly different), then to another IDT meeting. I also had many separate involvements with the Dietition, the Kitchen Manager, the RN on the floor, the Evening Nurse of the Day and each of the different PABs on each shift. There were about twenty-five different people (some several times) who had to be involved. It took a lot of perseverance on my part—just to get a bit of food!

And I forgot the psychiatrists that management sent me to, because they claimed that I had a problem with food. And then there was a three-month delay before I received the report from the psychiatrists. (The psychiatrist said it had been sent, management said they had not received it). Who had been sitting on it for three months? This report, when it came, was favourable to me.

There were complications along the way. Because I was so ill with the strokes, my maintenance needs were ignored—my teeth, eyes, gluten-free diet, yearly check of blood for colon cancer (for which I had surgery in 2004). My teeth needed major attention. The gluten-free diet is still under review, the eyes are back to having a yearly review on a condition of Closed Angle Glaucoma and Cataracts in both eyes. The colon cancer yearly blood tests have been resumed and have been clear for nine years.

After all of this and also having been through both six life-threatening illnesses *(pneumonia, infectious mononucleosis, infectious hepatitis, hysterectomy with complications, colon cancer, seven strokes)* and The Depression in my life, was I going to have to survive HUNGER?

Fortunately, the HUNGER problem has been solved with management coming to a snack solution, one of my nieces buying us a small refrigerator, and my purchasing of gluten-free products from a health store in Ontario.

Management is not mean with food—it is actually generous, just rather inefficient, with the problem very often being communication amongst staff or between resident and staff. Why doesn't the staff person ask the resident how she or he feels that person can be helped? We have brains, too.

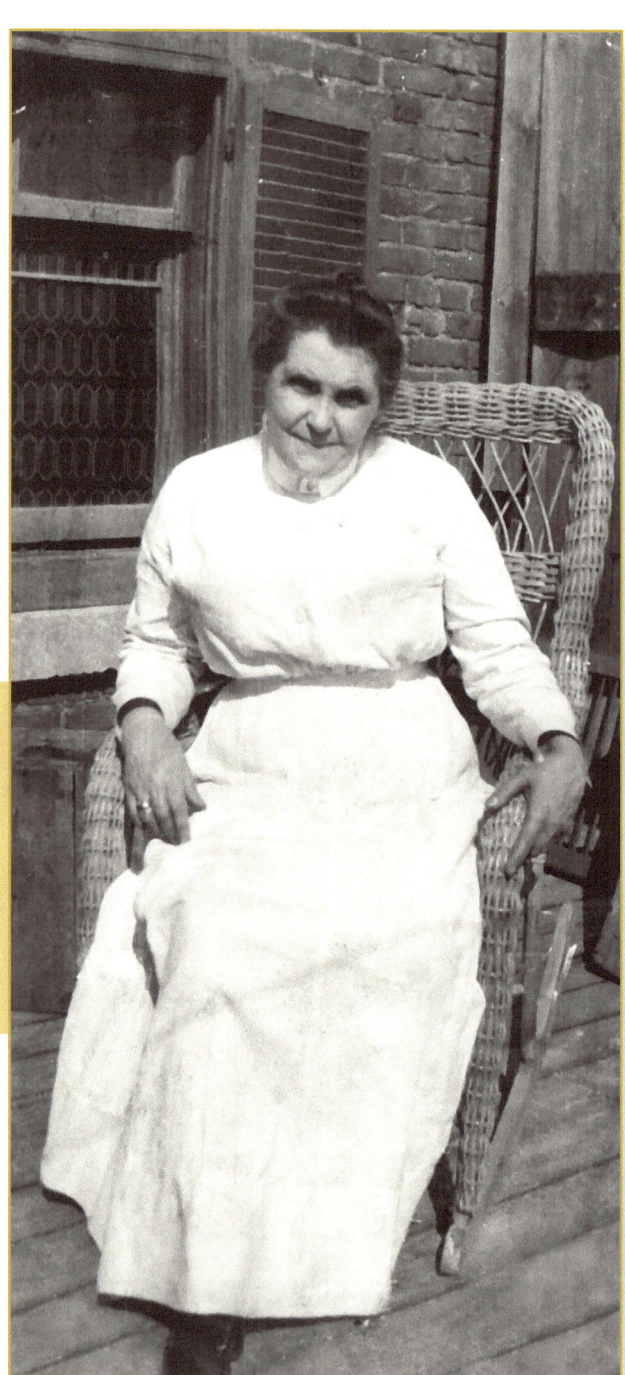

Grandma Hunter
in her midwifery dress

Nutrition and Cooking

Because I say that the HUNGER problem is solved, it doesn't mean that all the food problems are solved.

It would be nice to have some choice of the food. For instance—why must it be so many hard boiled eggs? What is the matter with a fried egg? a poached egg? a scrambled egg? When we were first admitted here we had scrambled eggs two or three times a week.

I asked the dietitian some time ago what happened to the scrambled eggs? She said 'it doesn't fit in with the workers' schedule'. What is the kitchen staff here for, but to help the residents? Is it really so tiring to scramble an egg? Is it really less tiring to hard boil an egg?

When I was a very little girl going to school, the priest used to come in every Friday morning to give us instruction. One Friday the lesson was on how to keep your husband. I went home that day and my mother gave us a lunch of white fish, white potatoes, white cauliflower with white sauce—and the meal was topped off with white ice cream. I immediately told my mother she would lose her husband, the priest said so!

Today here we had white fish, white potatoes, white ice cream. True, there were some orange carrots today—but I was inspired to relate about the boring white meals. Shouldn't the elderly have some input into the meals for the elderly?

So many meals in institutions are boring and uninspired. The elderly have taste buds too, and can appreciate good food presentation. One of the PABs told me that the menu hadn't been changed in 23 years—that I was wasting my time. But food is my passion—and it is so essential for good health and so many older people are so casual about their eating habits.

When I was first stricken with the seven strokes, I didn't want to live any more. I stopped eating many times, consciously.

I didn't want to die—but I wanted to be dead.

I had to watch my sister die in August 2010 because she couldn't eat any more, because all her systems had broken down, due to complications from Diabetes, and I finally had to agree with the doctors that she needed morphine, because of her terrible pain. It hurt me no end.

Friends had advised me to let her go as peacefully as possible. Family members questioned, suggested that people didn't realize how tough Charlotte was, that maybe she could ride this one out. She had won so many of life's battles. She was only three and a half pounds when born. As the closest one to her, I had to make the decision. I did consult religious and medical advisers and friends and relatives. It was unbearably difficult.

A year and a half before, she had been in a similar situation, this time in a medically induced coma in ICU for 6 days. The hospital had advised that we would have to consider removing the life support equipment. I had begged for two days for consideration. In that two days she came back herself. She thanked me many times in that period for helping her to enjoy that year and a half of life even though it was a difficult quality of life for her.

I had hoped I could do it again!

It always hurt me that though food is so important, it is taken so casually. I want very much to live now, just as long as I can.

When I was in the private nursing home, the administrative team heard of my love and expertise with food and asked me to teach two classes with food. So I taught two classes of residents. We all enjoyed the Banana Bread.

Residents look forward to meals. At this time, we don't even have a Residents' Committee here, so how can we have any input into food served to us? The Government has made a Residents' Committee the law. But we don't have a Residents' Committee. Why?

Management will tell us they have tried and nobody volunteered. I volunteered. They said one volunteer doesn't make a committee! I wonder why they don't try another approach to getting residents and families involved?

There are a few things that could be tried. A small office could be opened for an in-house ombudswoman/man for two hours per day where a resident or family member or friend or volunteer could stop in and voice a concern in a casual way or ask for answers about a troubling concern. A retired person or someone on light work might be interested.

It might be a way to show that the long-term care facility was interested in being a part of the community and that management genuinely wanted the residents and concerned families and friends to be involved in the running of their institution. I certainly don't feel they want my involvement. I very often feel that I am only here to help give management and staff a pay cheque.

I would also involve the other long-term facilities (6 or 7 of them I believe in the present amalgamation). Why do their Residents' Committees work—or do they?

Nobody seems to have any imagination here and that follows through to the food.

I am not stating that they are not kind or generous with the food—because they are—but maybe new involvement of interested persons could be quite wonderful. There are people here from so many different countries, could they be involved too? It could be fun to live here! We could try their cultural specialties.

I believe the kitchen needs recycling. I believe there needs to be in command someone who loves food and loves the elderly. I think they have neither at this time. There is far too much waste. I, personally, have put in my garbage $6,000 worth of food that I cannot eat, in the 5 years I have been in this Government Nursing Home.

I suggest Recommendations at the end of this book—but for the food—I wait to see what the Government recommends.

More Poetry

TABLE MANNERS

There go the table manners again
It would have been great to have them
As long as I lasted
But my hands tremble so much
That I must make a decision
The brain or the hands

The hands could be slowed
But the brain would also be slowed
Having lost my brain for a year and a half
When having seven strokes
In the first six months
Then a year in shock
Then having a miraculous recovery
   of my brain
I was not anxious to lose it again

So I made the choice
And sometimes sit on both hands
So it is good-bye to the table manners

Until I win big in the lottery
And can afford to have a cookery
Where food could be prepared in
   a suitable form
Without an abundance of finger food
To facilitate the return of my self esteem
And also the return of my
   table manners again

Where I ended up

I never thought that I would end up in an institution. But here I am, six years since I was found on the floor, near my bed.

The CLSC (local community health care center) worker found me. I wish I knew her name. I was unconscious for up to four hours. I should thank her for finding me and sending me to hospital. I came to in the ambulance. I don't remember much for the first 6 months except the terrible things that happened, and some of the funny ones that friends have told me about.

There was a 100 year old woman in the hospital room with me who used to pitch pieces of toast through the air to me as she said, "Somebody has to look after Carol."

I also got the name of Drama Queen at the hospital. I guess my life was a drama at that point.

I remember all the nights when I was being drugged and put out in the shed. It seemed every night for some time. There was one night when the ceiling fell on me and somehow I was responsible for that. That is how I remember it. I guess I was hallucinating.

I remember having a few brain scans. During one I was so agitated they could not proceed.

My friends tell me that I ate very little in hospital—mostly ice cream and yogurt. They said there was a kind dietitian who tried very hard to tempt me, but I only wanted the ice cream and yogurt.

In the first nursing home I remember seeing big fish coming out of the walls in the bedroom. And I remember seeing spiders running up the walls. Of course, there were none of these. Was it the drugs to treat the strokes? Was it the side effects of the mind altering drugs? I rarely have nightmares or hallucinations now—but then I am not on any mind altering drugs any more! I got off those as soon as I could.

Drugs & Things

I wonder if all the drugs that the elderly take are really necessary. I worked my way off all I could, but always with the knowledge and advice of the medical world. I am presently on just one small heart pill a day, and this is for an irregular heartbeat, they tell me. I do take one small Tylenol when in pain—very rarely.

I feel concern for the people who just sit there all day and don't react to much, except they holler. I don't know their medical conditions—so I can't judge. There are some who yell out for help, there are those who don't want to be washed, and then there are those who curse the workers. I feel very sorry for the PABs—I don't think that anybody who is trying to bring comfort to the residents should have to take that treatment.

I did hear two years ago that there would be another therapist here to work with cognitively impaired residents who were unable to react to much. I spoke to her and she said she was trained for that kind of work. I thought that was wonderful—but it never happened!

I think that most of the staff here are very kind to the residents. I wonder, though, if there could be someone who would listen to troubled residents and try to solve their problems. I guess what I am suggesting is an in-house ombudsperson. The hospitals have a Department of Pastoral Services. We do have a small Pastoral group of about four members.

I also wonder if the Government is moving towards turning this institution into a palliative care institution. It looks that way to me, as they keep raising the number of hours of nursing care needed for admission to this institution and so residents must be in a more difficult state to be accepted.

Some of the PABs who work here tell me about how their elderly are cared for in their home countries—at home! The

Government here, I hear on the radio, is now offering to pay 30% of homecare expenses. It really is a difficult and expensive time we live in. I, personally, have problems of food expenses.

Another problem that we have here is problem residents—difficult patients being admitted when I feel they should be in more specialised care facilities. I do not feel that our staff is trained to care for them or that the other residents can feel safe when they are mixed among them. I request that I be locked into my room every night because I am afraid to be beaten as I sleep. The resident I fear has now had an alarm installed in her room but with minimum staff at night I still am afraid of her coming into my room as I sleep.

My father was beaten as he lay in bed in long-term care. The nurse tried to choke him to death. His neck veins were blue, the finger indentations of his nurse were marked on his neck, his wrists were cut, he had a large bump on the back of his head and then she gave him a shot of tranquilizer. His room was on the 5th floor. His yelling was so loud that another nurse on the ground floor heard and came up and gave him another shot of tranquilizer.

My father was beaten 42 years ago—I still remember it as if it was yesterday. There was considerable loss of life when this institution suffered a fire several years ago—but I feel, by being locked in at night, that I would rather die of smoke inhalation, than of being beaten to death. My father did not die of the beating but the image of such suffering remains with me. He was in long-term care following a traffic accident. He had been standing on the sidewalk waiting for the traffic light to change when a car mounted the curb and hit him and he suffered many physical injuries including severe brain damage.

Another problem is that too many agency people are used here. I have just lived through trying to use the commode—it took one hour and ten minutes. It should have taken one regular staff person ten minutes, but instead it took two agency people one hour and ten minutes. Life for the elderly is not filled with joy! It could be much different if people cared for each other and even some of the smaller problems were solved.

Gluten-Free Diet For Gluten Sensitivity Disease

In 1994 doctors couldn't diagnose my problem, so I tried a dietitian. After many trials she was perplexed. She said, "Would you try a gluten-free diet?" I said, "Yes." She explained it to me and said I should try it for 2-3 weeks and let her know how I felt. I was so much better in just a few days. I was cooking for myself at the time.

When the 3 weeks were up she said, "Now you have to go back to a regular diet with bread every day and regular wheat products daily, and all the other forbidden foods, for at least 3 weeks." I didn't want to do that, but I started back. I lasted 3 days and I felt terribly sick. I accepted the fact that I needed to be gluten-free for the rest of my days and felt much better.

So for about 10 years, I lived gluten free. Then I was told by the hospital that they had tested me and I did not need to be gluten-free. However, they had tested me when mentally I wasn't with it from all the strokes.

So I went back on all the forbidden products, and the stomachaches and the gas and the diarrhea came back. The pain was so bad that I clung onto the bed sides and cried until the pain subsided. The terrible pains lasted for about 6 hours each time, sometimes on and off for about 4 days. The diarrhea (or loose stool, as they called it here) was with me for 3 years, alternating with constipation.

What I did not know was that the need to be gluten-free does not necessarily show up in a blood test if you are already on a gluten-free diet.

I had already decided to put myself on a gluten-free diet. As I now live in a long-term care facility, I was required to present a doctor's certificate stating that I needed a gluten-free diet—so I did not get it. I have had to find doctors who specialize in this and I have done so, but it takes months before you get an appointment, and then months before you get results. I waited for reports from blood tests and a gastroenterology test. Management was notified by written word and by telephone by the Gastroenterologist himself.

Meanwhile I have to find cash for gluten-free muffins and meat. They do supply me here with yogurt and ice cream and a basic diet of vegetables, fruits, and whatever else I can take from the tray. As I don't know what the ingredients are that they put in their dishes, I am afraid to try many of them. I did ask management last year if I could have half the money back that the Government advises me to pay every month and I would look after my meals. They just laughed!

I also did ask for an ingredient list—again it was no—impossible. It would be helpful to know what ingredients were in any particular dish that I am unfamiliar with. Sometimes I try a dish and suffer a very uncomfortable and painful stomach for 4 days. I think this is unkind and unnecessary. You must need to have a recipe for each dish prepared in the kitchen. Could I have a copy of each? Then I could make my own decision. As a result, I never take the soup or pudding as I do not know what is in either.

I have been losing weight with this up and down eating, so that is the reason I put myself back on the gluten-free diet and have since had no gastroenterology problems. But meanwhile, I have to find about $200 extra for food each month. Again, do we beg, borrow or steal?

When I came to this residence on May 20, 2008 I was questioned about my need to be gluten-free. I said it did not seem to be necessary any more because the hospital had tested me when I was a patient there from February to July 2007. Their test said that it was not necessary, yet on the admission sheet to the first long-term center, apparently it said that I needed to be gluten-free.

However, the first center never bothered with it. I was a patient there from July 2007 to May 2008. That is how it came to be on the second care center's admission sheet. Even though the first center never bothered with it, they still passed it on to the second center, and then they did not bother with it either.

When I was discharged from hospital my prognosis was "She will not recover. As you see her now, she will be until she dies." I waited to die from July 2007 to May 2008. Now, 6 years later, I wonder and cry when I realize that I was cut off all therapy and hope for 11 months.

What the hospital and the government did not know, or even guess, was that in the Summer of 2008 my brain would come back. I was so happy. Suddenly I could remember what our apartment looked like, what street our apartment looked out on, that my bedroom curtains were so beautiful, that my sister's paintings were so beautiful. I guess I had not appreciated how lucky I was. And now the beauty in my life is gone. Now I know that I must appreciate what I can do, and not dwell on what I cannot do.

I did prepare a very simplified description of the diet and gave it to the dietition with 10 copies—one for each of the kitchen staff—I never heard if it was circulated.

One wonders what the problem is in the kitchen. I wonder if there is any coordination. On Monday, November 14, 2011, why was I served two scrambled eggs for breakfast, which I finished at 11 a.m., and one hour later, at 12 noon, served two poached eggs for lunch? This is not the first time I have been served four eggs per day or even five, one day. It has happened about 4-5 times. I would suggest one kitchen worker be assigned to special diets.

I also wonder why kitchen and residents must exist so isolated from each other. Possibly if we could meet, we would feel more kindly disposed towards each other.

Some days, I don't even get a plate to eat my breakfast on. I eat it on a Kleenex. This is a little messy for cutting prunes or putting ketchup on a boiled egg or peanut butter on a muffin, which I have to order and pay for myself from a bakery in Ontario.

After 4½ years in this second health care long-term center, the institution has accepted the fact that I need a gluten-free diet. And I have been advised that Management will be supplying gluten-free muffins, cookies, and a variety of breads and cereals.

Management called an IDT (Inter Disciplinary Team) meeting and advised me that it was to be about me—so I went, having asked the President of the Residents' Committee to accompany me (as she has a close relative who must also follow a gluten-free diet). She was knowledgeable and advised the participants about my gluten-free needs.

The Montreal Gazette ran a two-page feature on Gluten Sensitivities. The Canadian Celiac Association ran a feature article on me in their Spring issue. The Suburban Newspaper and the Quebec Celiac News each ran an article on me concerning the difficulty in getting a gluten-free diet, and advising about the two gluten-free books I have written.

I guess that puts to sleep Management's first reaction to my complaint about food. They sent me to a psychiatrist! It should have been a gastroenterologist! I imagine they thought I was just having an idiosyncratic idea!

At the doctor's advice I have been in touch with the chemist who previously supplied all medication to this institution and have learned that none of the drugs that I take contain any gluten. Again on the doctor's advice I have consulted a dermatologist to learn if there was any complication. There

is not. The symptoms would be quite different. Those two possibilities are clear, therefore any gluten that reaches my body must come from the food.

I seem to have been legitimized and should have no further belly aches or diarrhea—if the kitchen pays attention to my needs.

Guess what?! The kitchen sometimes does very well by me and sometimes not. I really must scrutinize every plate that comes before me. I am still sometimes getting gluten-free and not gluten-free on the same plate, which cross-contaminates the gluten-free! I would say about 70% are now gluten-free.

December 13, 2012 was my 83rd Birthday. On December 14 the kitchen made a cake for me, which was very kind of them, but they made it with regular wheat flour, which is a No-No for anyone with Gluten Sensitivity Disease. A very brief bit of information would be helpful for anyone doing the cooking!

During the holidays of Christmas 2012/New Years 2013 I was served at least two pieces of cake, made again with wheat flour. At holiday time it could be understandable, but education is easily carried around with you.

The Canadian Celiac Association offered to conduct a presentation of the Gluten Free needs of anyone who was afflicted, and were refused! Does that make sense to you?

However, I refer you to my chapter on suicide.

I do appreciate that the Kitchen Staff must be asked to look out for me and I want to thank them. I want them to know why this is necessary. It is because I have lost 10 pounds in the last 20 months and two specialists have advised that I follow a Gluten-Free Diet.

An excerpt from
Essential Information For A Gluten-Free Diet

FOODS NOT TO EAT
• wheat • oats • barley • rye
and everything that contains those flours

The Reason Why I Am Asking For A Change Of Residence

*This book started as **Potty Training for an Octogenarian** and I was so pleased when I felt successful. I have since changed the name. But now which way will it go?*

One of my main caregivers decided that she would put me back into diapers. I was aghast, stunned, angry and not accepting. I was not incontinent and saw no reason for the change. At this point I had been wearing pull-ups for several months very successfully.

Her reason was that she would not have to help me to the commode at 10 a.m. She could then leave me in wet or dirty diapers from 8 a.m. when she washed me (not having put me on the commode at that time) until 2 p.m.

Remember, I am still wearing diapers at night, because I am in bed for 12-15 hours. I use the commode at 7:30 pm before I get into bed. At 11 p.m., a fresh heavy-duty diaper is put on. Most nights I do very little on the diaper and need to use the commode in the morning.

Before the potty training, I was wearing diapers round the clock for 4 years—from February 2007 to February 2011 and suffering with open sores on my buttocks. The sores were very painful and management tried many creams on them.

You change a baby when wet or dirty—but in seniors' residences there are those who seem to think it is ok to leave them wet or dirty for several hours. Before the pull-ups I was left from: 8 a.m. - 2 p.m., 2 p.m. - 7 p.m., 7 p.m. - 11 p.m. and 11 p.m. - 8 a.m.

The caregiver (PAB) tried several times to put the diaper on me instead of the pull-ups. The first time, I let her do it. I thought 'maybe she is tired'. The second time, I was just washed in bed. This time I rejected the diaper. She left me stark naked on the bed and went out to get the RN. The RN was surprised to see me naked, covered me with a towel, then told me it was just for today. What the reason was, I don't know.

Then there was the day that I was being helped from the commode, and again the PAB tried to put on a diaper. I rejected it and threw it on the bed. She flung the pull-ups after it and said, "You can get yourself dressed, I am not coming back into the room." I was left for an hour on the commode. I did get myself off the commode and onto the wheelchair—but not dressed. I wanted to be cleaned before I pulled up the pull-ups and the slacks. I had hurt my back a few weeks before and was unable to do the slacks myself.

I thought I was here to be helped!

And while sitting waiting for some help, my nephew came in and found me half dressed. This was embarrassing, humiliating. This is a man with whom I share a mutual respect. I don't think this is a good image of me or of this residence to be presented to the outside world.

Following this I requested a different caregiver and was refused. In the days following, the Evening Coordinator could see how upset I was and several times checked my blood pressure. It went up almost daily—125/70 (my normal count) to 145 and 153 and 168/77 and still a change of caregiver was refused. I have had seven strokes, I don't want an eighth.

During that period I did suffer a great deal of verbal abuse and threats. I had no witness, so I knew I would not be believed, so I did not even report them, but I have not forgotten them.

That Saturday morning as I lay in bed, crying and shaking, I was told all my bad qualities. I was told that I was the only one on the floor who knew what she was doing and yet I was the most troublesome. And on it went. I also was told that the floor was not run by the Evening Coordinator. One wonders why the Government thinks they are necessary. It is sometimes difficult to know who is the decision-maker.

I asked had anyone seen my mounting blood pressure in the report? It had not been seen. Why not? I believed it was there. I had seen it before my eyes on the machine, when it was taken.

So when I learned that nothing would be done on my behalf, I decided that I would have to either leave this residence, take my own life, or tell the truth about conditions here, in this instance. So I called the Residents' Committee President, and another Volunteer here, my Niece, my Lawyer and the Social Worker. I wonder why the government wants to keep us all in long-term care when some therapy and encouragement might help us to be less of a drain on society.

I am presently waiting for a response from the Social Worker about what residence might be more suitable for me, where the Resident's care would come first. I would be sad to leave the many good and dedicated, kind healthcare workers here, but unfortunately not all are so dedicated.

Meanwhile, on Monday morning, I did get a change of caregiver and life is more calm and pleasant with the present one. Yet I feel it comes at a price. My hands shake more, my legs are weaker than they used to be when I walk with the Physio, my sleep routine has been disturbed. I wake in the night and am unable to get back to sleep for 2-3 hours. I am back to the unsettling dreams. My scalp condition has worsened. I have to have treatment for it weekly for 6 weeks—at a cost to me. Yes, it has taken its toll.

I am still in pull-ups by day and diapers by night and the present caregiver will help me to the commode when I ask her to.

What would be the decision, on my behalf, another time, if the person in charge was not moved by my stroke history and the mounting of my blood pressure? What would have happened if the Evening Co-ordinator's advice was ignored? Was the action finally taken only because I involved so many people? And what about the poor souls who are not able to speak for themselves? In our hearts, are we satisfied with the quality of healthcare that we give to the vulnerable elderly in our care?

Am I safe in the care and absolute authority of someone whose core values are so different from my own?

August 26, 2011

Ten months later, I did hear from the Social Worker that a new residence was being made ready for intermediate care patients and that I was eligible. Then a few hours later the government said they wanted new tests done because the last ones were now a year old.

Forms were again filled out and returned and we wait again.

I feel badly about the PAB. She was so kind and efficient when I first came under her care, but when she returned from her two weeks of holidays, she seemed so different. She seemed mean and unkind and said terrible things to me and refused to do simple things that she had done before. But when my blood pressure rose so suddenly, I had to rebel. After all, I was the person who was here for care not for extra stress.

Now what happens to me, I do not know. When the Government informs us, we must then ask them many questions. Is there a physiotherapist in the intermediate care residence? Will I get a gluten-free diet? Etc.

July 12, 2012

The Government did notify us—that there was no room for me. They had filled the new building with people waiting in hospital and it would be a very long time before they had room for me.

September 2, 2012

The Social Worker of our institution did inquire whether the intermediate care center was serviced by either a physiotherapist or a dietitian. The answer was NO! Where would be the help for me? I need both, if I am not to be a drain on society forever!

Nursing Care

I have seen three qualities of nursing care—excellent care, sloppy care and dangerous care.

Excellent Care is given by nurses who see a need for care and give it. They take the patient and the job seriously.

Sloppy Care is when a nurse says, "I'll be back later," and you never see her again.

Dangerous Care is when a nurse gives the wrong medication.

I was a victim, or rather an attempted victim, of the Dangerous Care category. A nurse gave me my one small pill of the day, which was normal and prescribed. Then she came back and tried to give me three more. I said they were not mine. She said the doctor had ordered them for me. "And what doctor is that?" I asked. "You tell that doctor to come right here and tell me what the pills are and what they are for."

What happens to the cognitively impaired patients who cannot fight for themselves?

It strikes me that nurses should know what they are doing. The nurse was so aggressive that had a PAB not been in the room to back me up, I believe the nurse would have tried to force them down my throat. A group of PABs on the floor insisted that I report the incident to management, which I did, and was told by management that they would get back to me. That was about 4 years ago. I never heard another word!

Sloppy Care was what management gave me in this instance. It did not build confidence with the resident (me).

A good nurse would have gone through her files and discovered where the three pills were missing, and a good supervisor would have been very concerned. As so many things are ignored here, this was just another one. The Montreal Coroner is talking about asking for death certificates to state cause of death in nursing homes! One wonders!

And yet, I have seen very good care, very professional, even very tender care, as if the nurse cared about what she was doing, and to whom. In this instance, she was washing out my eye. It was 11 p.m. but she was not rushed or rattled as they sometimes are at the end of a shift. She was just doing her work in a professional manner, and the only adjective I could use to describe it was 'tender'.

Another instance of good care was when I was refusing to eat. I saw no point in carrying on with living. I was so distressed with my lot in life. I was unable to do anything for myself. So I stopped eating and drinking. I thought '3-5 days—that should do it!' The nurse said "If you could make a choice, what would you like to eat?" I thought 'she will never find it', so I asked for cheesecake. Well, she found it! And she stood there beside my bed, and she fed it to me because I was shaking so much. Then she gave me a very small lecture on how "we needed to fight this on a full stomach, not an empty one." As I can usually see the funny side, I started eating again.

Then there was a nurse to whom you could always bring your troubles. She never demeaned you. She would listen. She didn't always agree with you, but you got a hearing. If it was in her power to help, she did.

Guess what? These examples of an Excellent Nurse are all the same person! She is retired now, and I miss her. She will recognize herself if she reads this. She is the only one who ever had to feed me cheesecake!

There were two Excellent Nurses at the first long-term care facility—just to state that there was more than one Excellent Nurse.

One of the purposes in writing this book is to try to bring back motivation to those who work in the healthcare field. I believe they start in this line of work because they are motivated, but somewhere the motivation slackens. Is it the pressure of work? Is it because they are not always appreciated? It would be pretty awful without them. So the next time you are cursed at, try to let it run off your back, and remember we don't all feel that way.

PABs

There are PABs here from many countries in the world, and most are very good. What I especially like is that they are very kind. They come from The Philippines, Jamaica, Trinidad, The Bahamas, Barbados, Bermuda, St. Vincent, South Africa, Haiti, China, Vietnam, Kenya, Nigeria, Cameroon, Pakistan, Grenada, Panama, etc.

My life would be much more difficult without them. If there is something missing on my tray, they will try to get it for me. I am learning about their countries as I get washed and dressed. I also learn about their lives here. One PAB came into my room when another one was working with me and said, "How come you know more about her than you know about me?" "So tell me your story," I replied.

I wish I had as good a relationship with the Kitchen staff as I do with the PABs and the Cleaning staff, but somehow the Kitchen seems to keep its distance from me. This hurts me, as food is my passion, and with as much catering experience as I have had in my career, it seems very odd to me that the Kitchen here is so unapproachable.

I feel for all who come so far from foreign countries to care for our old and ill. They leave their families and friends and come to a new environment and mostly are so good tempered and kind. I do admire them.

Religion

This long-term care facility was originally started by the Roman Catholic Church and remains fundamentally RC. However, not all residents belong to that religion, many from other religions are welcomed. There is a Catholic Chaplain here and Mass is held Wednesday, Friday, Sunday and is well attended. There is a small Pastoral Group which is quite active.

Auxiliary

There is an Auxiliary here whose members bring residents down on the elevator to Mass, serve goodies on a Friday, donate Christmas and Birthday gifts, operate the Tuck Shop, plan and operate several functions.

Medical Care

There are three physicians who cover the medical care needed here by the residents. If specialists or hospitalization may be necessary, residents may be sent out.

Therapy

A Physiotherapist and an Occupational Therapist are on staff here.

Foot Care

There is a Foot Care Specialist available about once a month.

Hair Salon

There is a Hairdresser on the premises in the Salon three days a week.

Nutrition

There is a Dietition on staff here.

IDT—Inter Disciplinary Team

There are meetings held with each resident yearly, which include management and department heads. They are supposedly to listen to any problems or complaints of the resident. It has been my experience that management shows a confrontational approach to any problem, and is mainly interested in protecting their own jobs. They are not really interested in solving my problems.

I have been in this institution five years and have attended four of these meetings. There were four different people chairing the meetings. One was welcoming, cheerful and kind. Another was stiff and frozen. Another was sometimes cheerful, sometimes very firm. Another was casual. In each case the result was the same—we had to wait outside the door for an unreasonable time even though we had been advised to be on time—and then the results were zilch.

In my case, their solution was to send me to a psychiatrist! Their food did not agree with me—so it must have been in my head! It should have been a gastroenterologist!

Actually I saw two psychiatrists—one was a doctor just finishing his Residency in Psychiatry and the other was a Staff Psychiatrist in the Psycho-Geriatric Department. They seemed to agree that I was pretty much o.k. and should have more Physiotherapy, which I had requested and did not receive.

I really feel there is no point in appearing at any meeting with management, as there is no meeting of minds. And while I look forward to the establishment of a Residents' Committee, I wonder if it has any hope of success!

I have always felt that management treats me as just another one of their poor Alzheimer's patients. It does not matter at all to management that in my fifties I received a Certificate in Management in Health and Social Services from McGill University. At this time I was employed as Executive Secretary to the Director General of a long-term centre in Montreal, and at the same time served as Union Representative on its Board of Directors (voted in by union members), and also was employed by the Medical Director in his private practice on Saturdays. I would appreciate being treated as the intelligent professional woman that I am.

Residents' Committee

The Residents' Committee, which was non-existent for the first few years that I was here, has been rejuvenated, and it seems to be working well. We do not hear of personal solutions, so I can only refer to my own. The President has helped me in two instances. They have regular meetings and seem to complain about the food.

Coordinators

There seems to be a Coordinator on each shift, who must also be the only authority for residents to appeal to. Sometimes we are just told he/she is too busy for our problem—take it up with the next shift. The next shift says it did not happen on my shift, take it up with the correct shift and the correct person. And so you give up and another problem just gets swept under the carpet!

Ombudsperson

It seems to me that there are three groups assigned to help the residents. In this time of amalgamation could we not combine them? Could we have an in-house ombudsperson with authority and decision-making power who could listen and solve problems and possibly refer major problems to a committee of three—made up of one from each group?

It strikes me that facing seven members of the IDT can be overwhelming for a resident to face when thay have a problem.

Laundry

The laundry service to the residents is included in the monthly fee. When we first came here, it was excellent. Laundry was returned every Monday and Thursday evening and nothing was ever ruined or lost. Through the last few years so much has been lost, so much has been ruined, that I would advise anyone who is able, to take their laundry home and do it there, to do that.

I don't have a home any more. We had to break up our home as my sister and I were both unable to care for ourselves any more.

One lovely long black skirt is now pale beige-grey and another long navy and grey skirt is now beige. I guess someone pushed the javel button. A top that used to be navy blue is now beige. Besides that, javel hurts delicate skin—so I am unable to wear them.

A beautiful nightgown has long since disappeared. One of the staff said, "Now that you know what they are using it for, do you really want it back?"

I can't afford to replace the clothing items ruined or lost, and management says they take no responsibility. I guess there is no point in replacing them even if I had the money, because they will only be ruined again.

For several days, I wore a sign on my chest saying:

TOPLESS SOON

One person's comment was "Promises—promises!"

It's funny—but it isn't funny. I have always cared how I look. But now there are so many articles of clothing gone or ruined that I don't even list them any more. But my choice of what to wear is certainly limited.

Maintenance & Cleaning

Maintenance and cleaning personnel are agreeable. I think it would be preferable if garbage could be picked up twice a day instead of once. Sometimes the PABs will take it out, but some of them just say, "It's not my job." Sometimes when overflowing I have been refused!

It would be pleasant to have a bench or a couple of chairs outside the front door, year round, as was the custom until this year. My friends often come to visit and take me out for some fresh air. In the off-season they must go inside and beg for 2 chairs – some people permit that—others are quite rude to them.

Approximately two years ago I asked could I have one wall in my bedroom painted because there were several spots without paint and when I have visitors they have to face that wall. I was told no—because it was planned that all the rooms would be painted very shortly. They have not been touched in the five years since I have been in this room, and it was not done when I moved in!

The curtains are finished in my room. The lining is ripped. No air is allowed in if the curtain is pulled. When they are replaced, because of the architecture of the building and the opening of the windows, management should consider blinds that pull up and down, not side to side. Then a resident could have some fresh air in the summer.

Another thing that needs consideration is the toilets. The one that joins my room is too low and crooked—no wonder the person who shares the bathroom with me fell off the toilet and broke her ankle. I tried using the toilet for one week and found it unsafe and uncomfortable. I must now use a commode in my bedroom with various people coming into my bedroom. It is crude, it is rude, it is horrible. Because we are old and ill and need help, it seems alright to treat the elderly without respect or dignity. There is a reason why it is the law to have ventilation in the bathrooms. A bedroom should not be used as a bathroom. It can be very smelly and embarrassing. For sanitary reasons the bathroom should be divided in two, one side for each resident.

Teeth

My teeth were in bad shape when I felt brave enough to have them looked at. Eight teeth needed extractions and I needed a full set of dentures. The Neurologist advised 'not to let anybody talk me into having a general anaesthetic, because my brain had had enough punishment'. So it was decided that one dentist would do the extractions and another the dentures, each being an expert in their field.

It took close to two years to have the work completed. I said when I had the new teeth I would look for a new life with a new smile. I have not looked yet, because it takes longer to get accustomed to my new image than I expected.

Glasses

In the Spring of 2009, I realized that I needed the lenses in my glasses checked. After ten years with the old frames I would have liked new frames but there was not money for that. It would have cost money to go out to an optometrist, so I took the Yellow Pages and looked for one in the area who made house calls. She charged a very reasonable price and brought the necessary equipment.

Within two weeks, my sight was adjusted. But again, I had to make the initial request and follow through with the glasses and the teeth. I tell you this because I want to show that I seem to be doing more and more as time goes on. And I want to. But why did I have to lose 11 months by being denied any therapy and hope by being given such a poor prognosis? I wash my own teeth, I wash my glasses and I wash some of my unmentionables and blouses. I wash three-quarters of myself (which is all I can reach). I can't get out of bed by myself, but I am trying to do more all the time. I think we should be encouraged to do as much as we can, instead of being left with no hope.

Walking

Yesterday I said I could not get out of bed on my own, today I did it!

Of course the PAB was with me raising and lowering the bed sides as I needed them. But I actually raised myself and stood by myself and sat by myself in the wheelchair. As I keep saying, I should not have been written off so readily. I certainly do not think that I am all recovered and able to look after myself, but I think that it is time that hope was given to the elderly, and therapy!

I do receive some therapy at this time, but it is called Maintenance Therapy. It is three times a week for about thirty minutes of walking on the double bars and about twenty minutes of putting on and off the ankle supports and shoes and socks by the therapist, because my left foot has gone crooked. I would like a more varied exercise program and more often—preferably daily. The therapist here says she is responsible for all the residents—that is 134 residents in this institution. When she is on holiday or attending meetings there is nobody to replace her—so we get no therapy. She needs her holidays, but we need our therapy. We do get some exercises to do on the off days.

The therapist should be replaced when on holiday. In fact the therapist should have an assistant all the time. We could all be in better shape.

I hope that I will walk normally again—but it is not looking hopeful at this time. However, it is in the lap of the gods!

But then who expected me to talk clearly or to write and publish two books and this third one in the works right now?

All I want is a chance to reach my full potential in my present state. What I want for all the elderly and injured is hope and encouragement. Please don't take that away from us.

The Computer

Now that I can write again, I wonder what I would like to do?

The thing that I would like to do is finish my Gluten Free Soup Cookbook that I had been working on when I had the first stroke. But how would I do that? My hands were not very good, my brain was not very wonderful. I had not typed in two years. I did not have a machine (the hospital had told my family that my useful days were over, so I had given away all my machines—from bread maker to computer).

I thought that perhaps if I could find a Word Processor I could cope. Well, of course, the world was past that. My niece, Cathy, called and asked if I would like to have her late Mother's laptop. I was petrified. I did not know how to turn any computer on or off. Everything had been jumbled in my brain by the strokes.

Had anyone saved the disks with backups on them or was the whole thing gone? Were the pictures gone? Some of the nieces had packed up the apartment. Had they saved or pitched? Fortunately, they had saved.

The nieces gave me the confidence that I was smart enough, that I could pick it up again. Well, I did, but it was not like bouncing back, it was more like crawling back! And many people helped me.

And I went on to finish and publish the Gluten Free Soup Book, which is now for sale on Amazon, along with a Gluten Free Dinner Book which I have also since prepared. And I am currently working on this book.

This is to prove that, even if the experts write you off—maybe you should not have been written off! I firmly believe I should have been given more therapy all along, instead of being dumped and just written off. I should have been recycled. Instead of that I am having to recycle myself.

Itchy Skin & Bloody Nose

Is it because of the dry air in the building? Or something in the food? Or the javel in the wash water? Or the soap or the detergent? Or the mattress or the pillows? Or the one small pill a day that I take? Or something else?

I have suffered from such itch since I moved to this room five years ago, and mostly in bed at night. I would so like to find a solution. Some nights I am jumping out of my skin with the itch and sleep very poorly, and other nights I sleep like a baby.

Do I need a psychiatrist, a humidifier, a new mattress, a change in diet, or what?

And then there is the bloody nose every morning and night. I guess the only answer for that is a humidifier. But the room is so small and a quiet humidifier is so expensive.

These are my problems, and probably another person would not have the same problems. I tell you so that the reader will realize that life goes on in a long-term care facility, and some problems are easier to solve than others.

A Sad Moment

A sad moment in a resident's life comes when a PAB who has been your caregiver for two years is transferred to another floor. Her going away gift to me was a pair of pull-ups. Nice touch—don't you think? It is nice to know that somebody has faith in me.

Room Safety

There is a lock on each door and a resident can ask for the key. I never felt that was necessary for most of the time I was here until one of the residents started going into other rooms and lifting things and stuffing them into her bra. Usually the staff retrieve the articles when preparing her for bed.

I believe the staff are honest. I have lost many pieces of clothing but I believe the problem arises when the clothes go down to the laundry and are returned to the wrong room. If the clothes are returned to the room of a cognitively impaired person, she will not even know it. When she dies the clothes are disposed of. So it is just inefficiency again, not stealing.

And yes, my clothes all have my name on them. I do lock my door now when I am not in my room.

Outside Physicians' Appointments

A difficult day in a resident's life is when a resident must go out for a doctor's appointment. It can be very exhausting. One recent one, for me, took five hours. This is a long day for a person who is not well in the first place.

- First there was a 35 minute wait for a Medi-Car (it was late)
- Then to find the way in the hospital
- Registering in the Clinic
- A 1 hour wait for the doctor
- Only to be interviewed by a medical student for another hour
- Wait for the student to update the doctor
- Talk to the doctor for a few minutes
- Go to another room for a blood test
- Phone the Medi-Car for a pick-up
- Wait 30 minutes for car
- Return drive—25 minutes
- 5 hours in all

Entertainment

There are many activities available for the residents—movies, bingo, happy hour, shuffleboard, bowling, discussion groups, music, singing, parties, mental aerobics, outings such as drives and picnics, barbeques. They are all well attended. I, myself, am not a joiner or a bingo or party person. I prefer working on the computer, entertaining by telephone, or in person, or keeping in touch by letter, or reading, or going out for fresh air, or exercising my legs in the gym.

Sum Up

I want to sum up my own feelings of my last six years in the healthcare system. So perhaps you would bear with me.

The six months in the hospital were frightening, overwhelming. They kept me alive, and they did give me some physiotherapy. I was walking with a walker on flat floors and even up 5-10 stairs with just holding on to the handrail. That was after the first stroke. Then I had six more, and they sent me out with a terrible prognosis. I would get no better! *"As you see her now, she will be until she dies."*

Well, they didn't know who they were talking about!

Eleven months we were in the first long-term care facility, my sister and I. I was in a very nervous state there, on mind-altering drugs. When I got off them I started to improve. Two of the nurses were very kind to me, also one or two of the PABs. Most of the PABs left a lot to be desired. They would put me to bed, leave everything out of my reach, go out for supper, and then I would cry for an hour until they returned. Management gave me no therapy. They had nice sitting out areas which I was able to use. Their bath areas have left me traumatized. It was 5 years in the second centre before I was able to take regular showers with any kind of peace. Their manager was very sympathetic and kind, compassionate, I guess you would describe her. All told it was a very mixed bag, and I was not sorry to leave.

And now I am in the current long-term care facility. The feeling here is kind and friendly, though I have had no ice cream for two days now, and the yogurt seems to have run out, too. Those are two things I can eat when they don't serve me any gluten free food. I did have a very nice lunch yesterday. I even sent a note to the kitchen saying so. Today the lunch was delicious, so a note again.

There is currently a meeting going on downstairs of the revitalized Residents'

Committee. I am not there. I decided not to attend, because there is 'no meeting of minds' between management and me. However, I am not planning to move out, until I win the Lotto!

My overall feeling is that I am pleased that there are so many good people willing to work so hard in the healthcare field here in Montreal, Quebec. I wish that some or all of my following recommendations could be considered.

I wish that somehow residents' conditions could be grouped together so that we would not be such a mixed group. We have yelling with foul language by the hour. It is rather depressing, and yet I do know that when I was having the strokes in the hospital I was making rather a lot of noise myself. I do not know how to improve the situation because residents do come here in one condition, which will probably change, and staff cannot keep on popping them around. I wish for a few soundproof rooms.

Possibly my writing this book will highlight some of the problems I have experienced. I hope it does not make things worse. It is meant to improve the situation. As I have been both Staff and Resident (5 years as each) I hope that my experiences can help to make life more pleasant and secure for the elderly. Surely some paint and blinds for the residents' rooms should be possible. It would tell the residents that we are as important as the public rooms, where the floors are always so shiny.

My Ancestors & The Montreal Community

My relatives have done so much for the Montreal Community, both in the health care and educational fields. I would like the reader to know that when I speak for the seniors it is because I feel I know them so well.

SARA P. TANSEY, my aunt. She was for almost half a century Founding Director of The Montreal Convalescent Hospital. With a group, she started the Hospital. Most of her adult life was given to it. She was totally dedicated to the well-being of her patients. Her photograph appears on page 11 (as a child), on page 55 (as a young woman) and on page 56 (in later life).

ROSEMARY TANSEY, my aunt. She was an RN with a Masters Degree. She served for many years as Chief Admissions Officer at The Montreal Convalescent Hospital, after training in and being employed in New York. Photos on page 11 (as a child) and page 56.

MICHAEL TANSEY, my father. He was a Financial Campaign Director for many institutions, mainly in the Healthcare and Educational fields. He was associated with at least ten hospitals in Montreal and one in Quebec City. He was also connected with a University and several educational institutions here in Quebec. Photos pages i, iii, 11.

JAMES HUNTER, my grandfather on my mother's side. He was a Minister in the Presbyterian Church in Scotland with a Masters Degree from a University in Scotland. When he came to Montreal he gave up the Ministry and opened his own school here to prepare boys for McGill University. His fees were fifty cents an hour —not a fortune. Photos pages 11, 51.

CHARLOTTE (SUTHERLAND) HUNTER, my grandmother. Grandma was a midwife and assisted many Montreal doctors and many mothers in the delivery of their babies, besides having six of her own. She was the only grandparent I knew. My grandfathers were both dead before I was born, the other grandmother died when I was two. Photos pages 11, 12, 16, 52.

CHARLOTTE HUNTER TANSEY, my sister. Charlotte had five degrees, three of which were Honorary Doctorates, from different universities—Concordia University, Bishop's University, and one in Vermont, USA. She was a Founding Director of the Thomas More Institute and was with them for sixty-four years. She retired after 18 years as President. Charlotte was totally dedicated to her students. She was also, as editor, involved in many educational books and government projects. Photos pages 12, 13, 57.

JAMES HUNTER (Son Of James Hunter and Charlotte Sutherland Hunter), my uncle. My Uncle Jim was a Pharmacist for the better part of his life right here in Montreal. Photo page 11, 58.

WILLIAM F. SUMMERS, my brother-in-law. Bill had a doctorate in Geography. He died recently at 93 years old. He lived most of his life in Newfoundland, but he also studied and taught at McGill University for several years. He had lately been honoured by Memorial University in Newfoundland, by having a seminar room named after him, because he was the first Head of the Geography Department, and he held that position for several years. Photo page 60.

MARY (TANSEY) SUMMERS, my sister. Mary had two university degrees, eight children and, with her husband Bill, wrote a textbook on the Geography of Newfoundland. She also wrote a mystery novel set in Edinburgh, Scotland. She worked in Medical Research here in Montreal before moving to Newfoundland. Photos pages 12, 13, 60.

CATHY TANSEY, my niece. Two years ago Cathy achieved her PhD in Medical Research. She has been working in this field for several years—10 years in Montreal, 20 years in Toronto and again the last 2 years in Montreal. Photos pages i, 56, 59.

BARBARA (TANSEY) COOPER, my sister. Though she has lived in England since 1952, she is a writer with a degree from the University of Montreal, and has written and published six Historical Romance Novels, five of which are set in early Quebec—mostly in Montreal and the surrounding area. These novels have been translated into French, Spanish, Portuguese, Swedish, Norwegian and sold in these countries—so that Quebec is getting good publicity across the world. Barbara's area of expertise has always been early Quebec since when she first wrote **THE CHOOSING** about the King of France giving, as his dowry to the girls of France, the boat fare to travel to marry settlers in the New World. His dowry was an ox and a cow, two pigs, a pair of chickens, two barrels of salted meat, and eleven crowns in money. Barbara's books may still be available in libraries in Montreal, in large print. Photos pages 12, 13, 61.

I list these members of my family because they are the ones who have given their working lives to health care and education here in Quebec. There are many others in the family who are in business, or lawyers.

I want the reader to know that we have given much of our lives to Montreal and Quebec and we have every right to be here, and to be served in our language in the healthcare and educational institutions that we helped to create and make possible for future generations.

All of us get along very well with people of other languages if left in peace. My belief is that children should attend school half day in English, half day in French, and in no time the whole population would be bilingual. No more problems. And could we start on being more considerate to the seniors who have made all this possible?

Montreal is a beautiful city and I am grateful to its Founding Nations—the French, the Irish, the Scots and the English—along with all the newer citizens from farflung parts of the world. Each culture has provided essential aspects that join together to make a wonderful whole.

This book is my contribution. It is my hope that it will help improve long-term care for seniors. It is based on my experience as both Staff and Resident in healthcare facilities for seniors in Montreal.

Prognosis for a Septuagenarian/Octogenarian

James Hunter—Grandfather

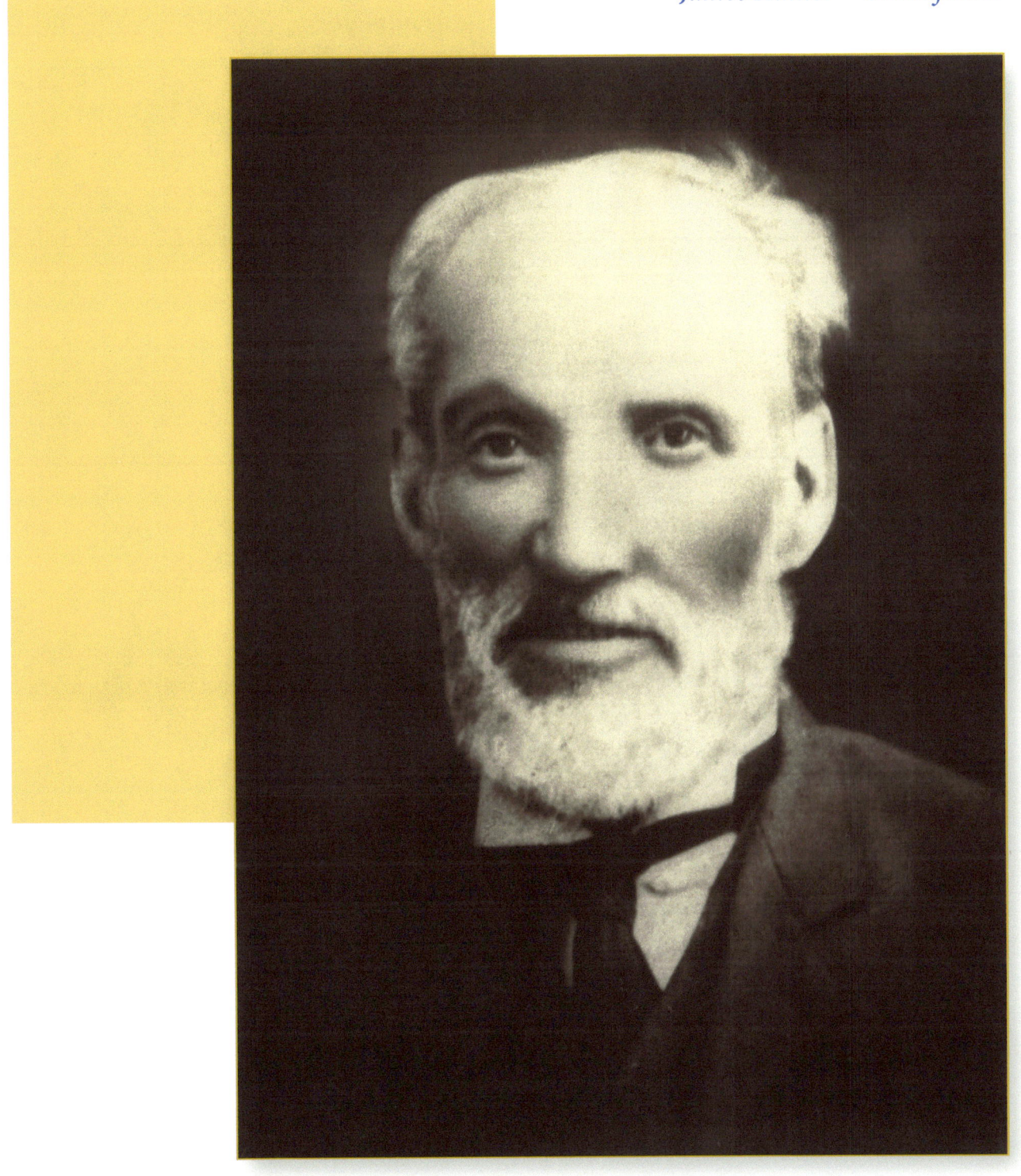

*Charlotte (Sutherland) Hunter
—Grandmother*

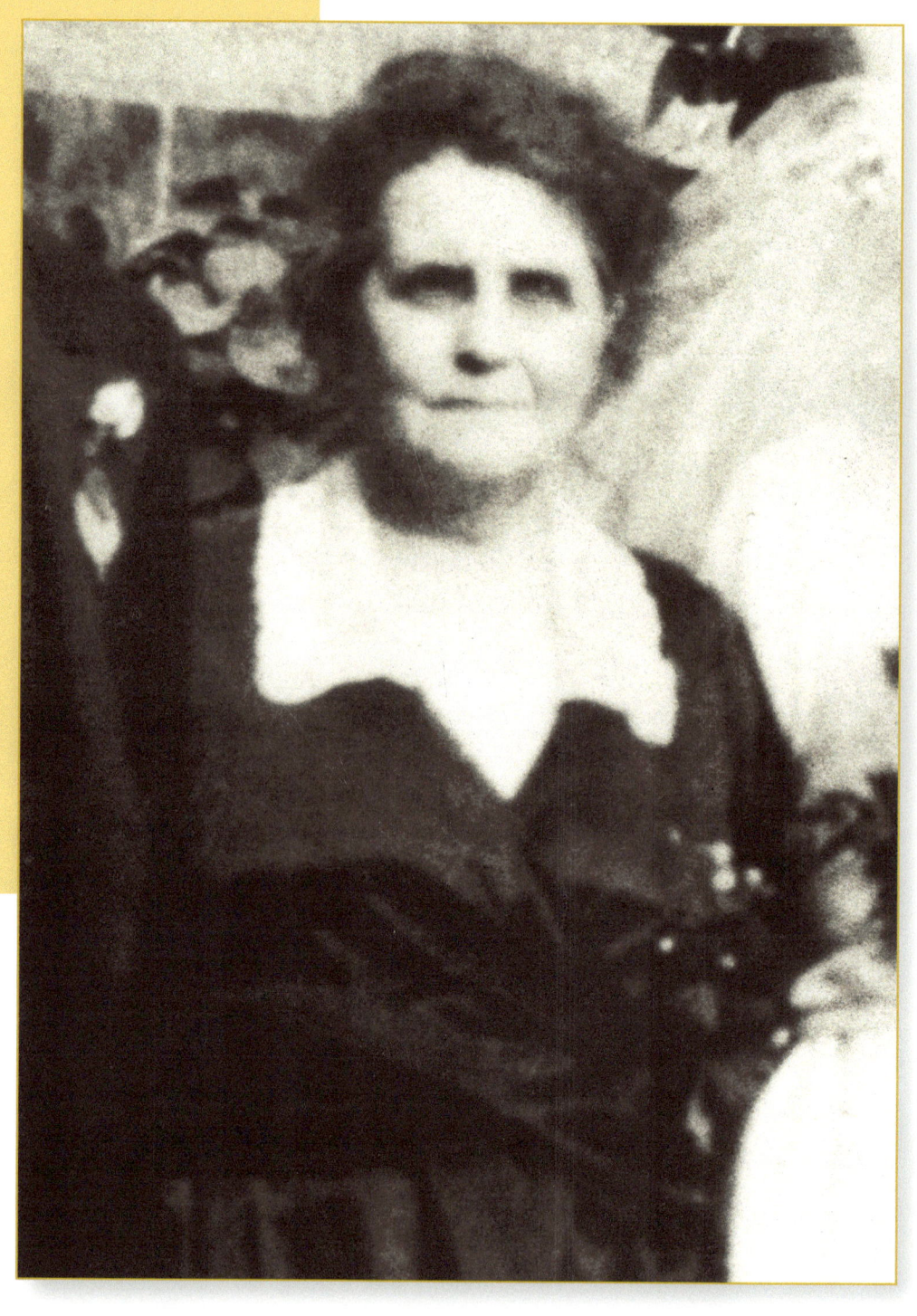

*Mary Elizabeth (Coffey) Tansey
—Grandmother*

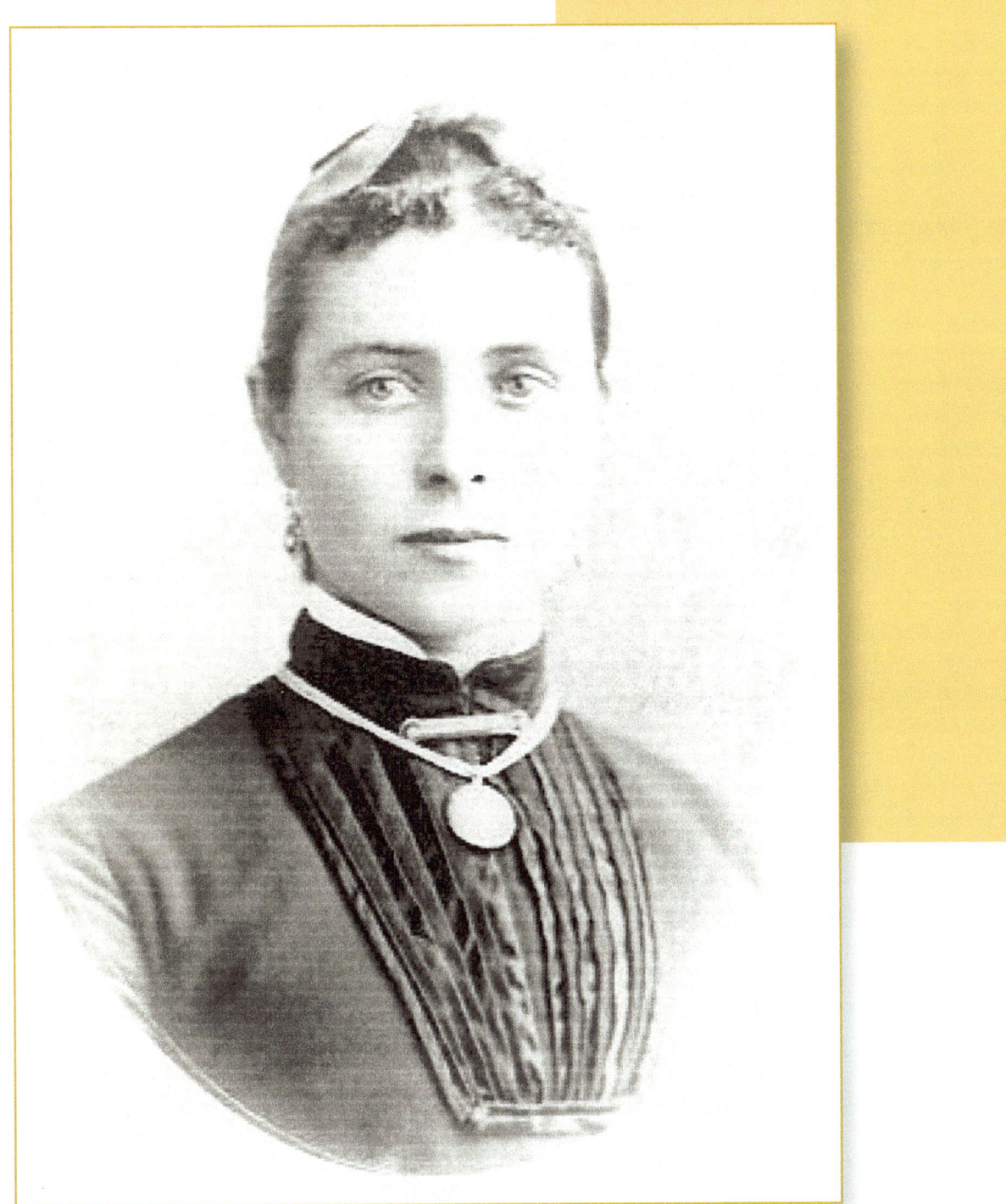

*Timothy Peter Tansey
—Grandfather*

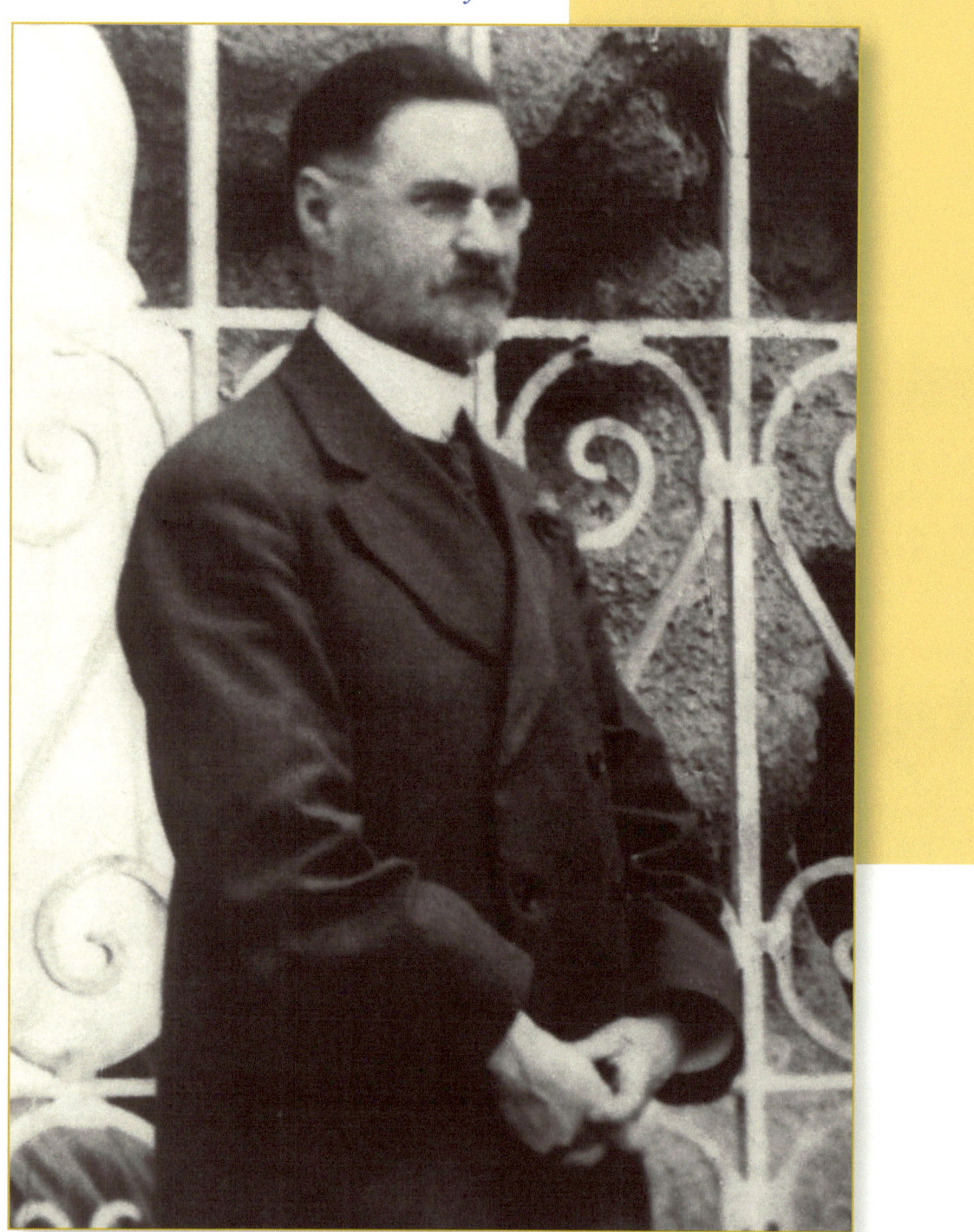

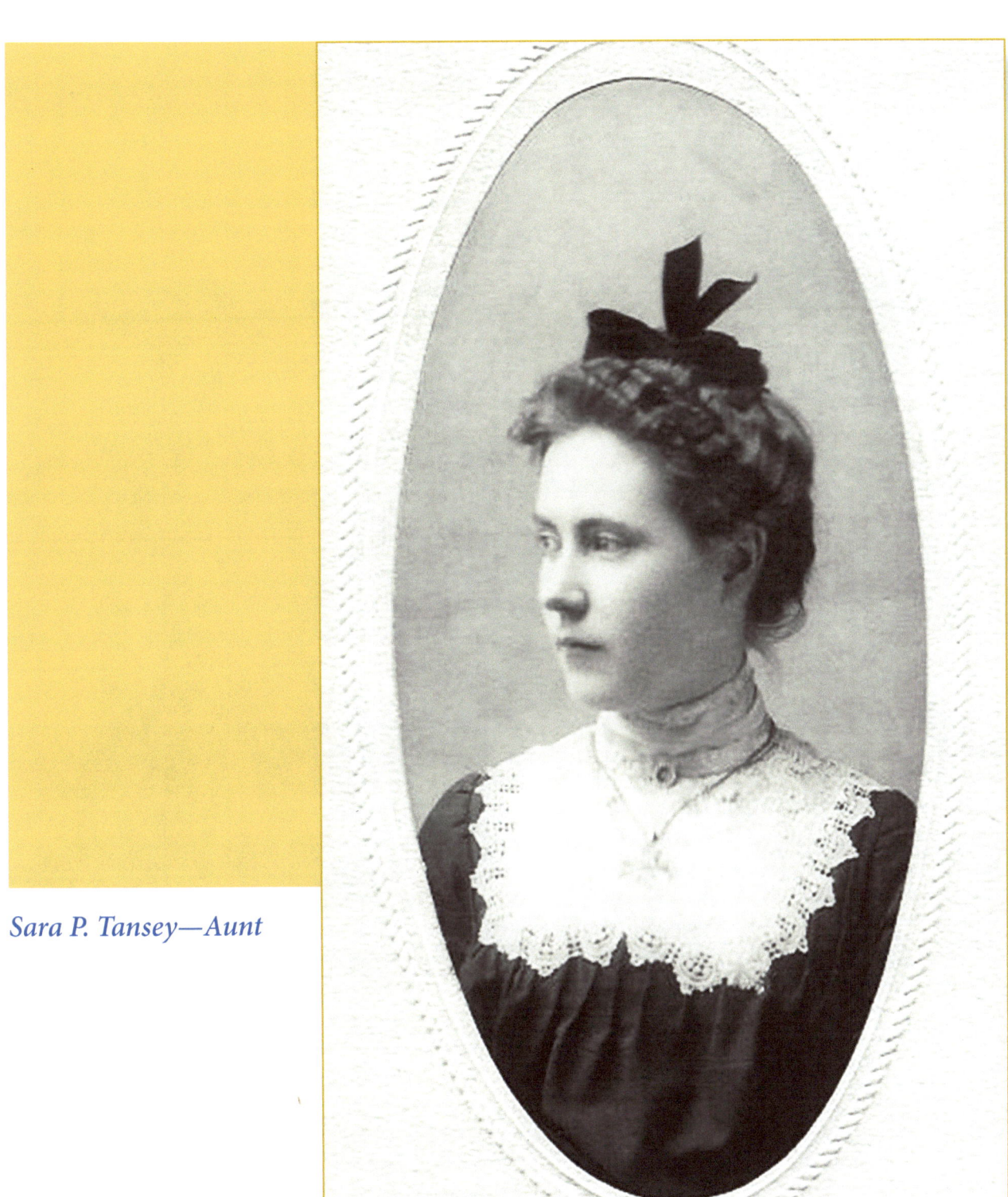

Sara P. Tansey—Aunt

Margaret, Sara & Rosemary Tansey
with *Cathy Tansey, Timothy Summers,
Patricia Tansey & Nicholas Summers*

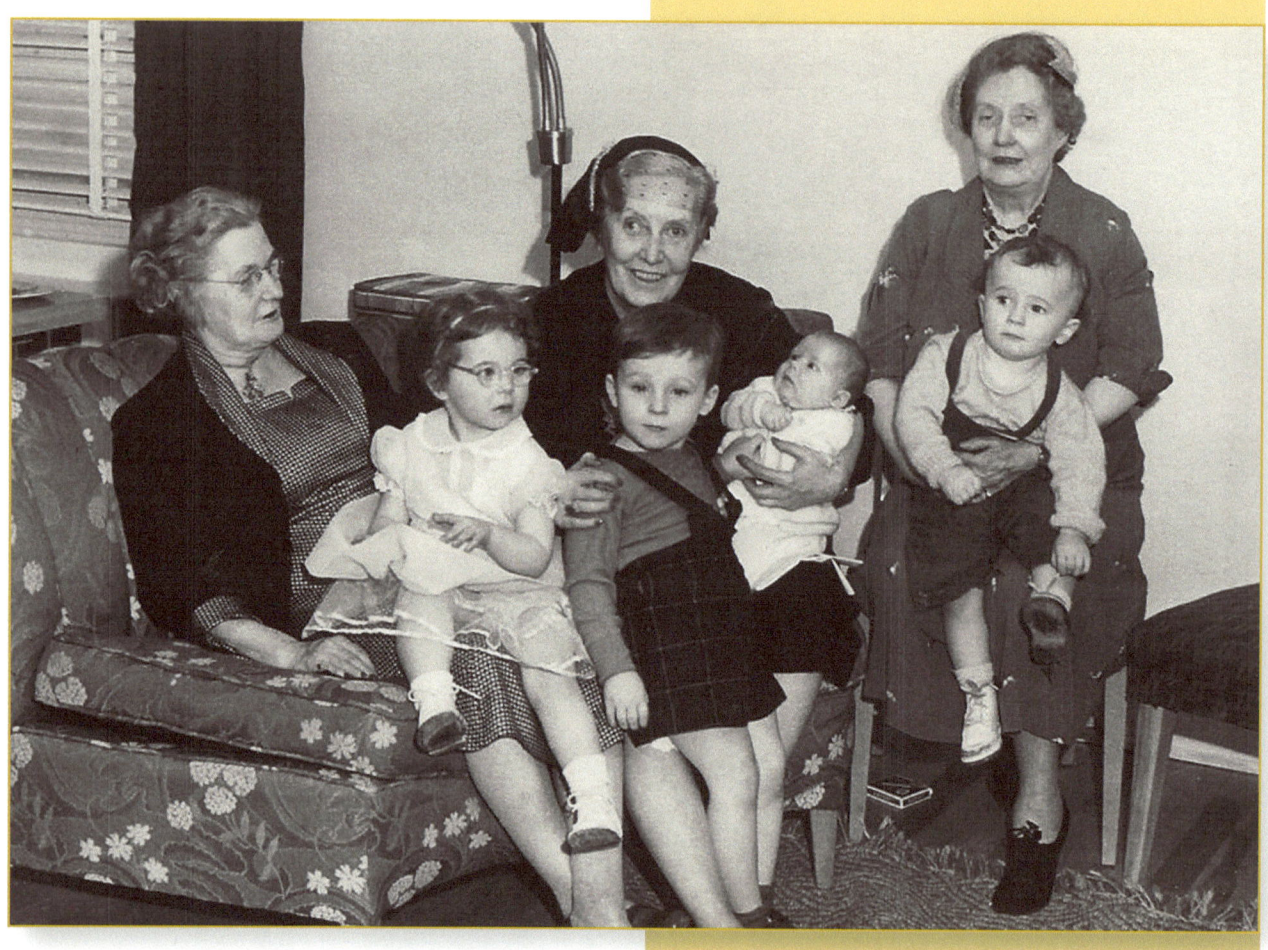

Charlotte Hunter Tansey—Sister

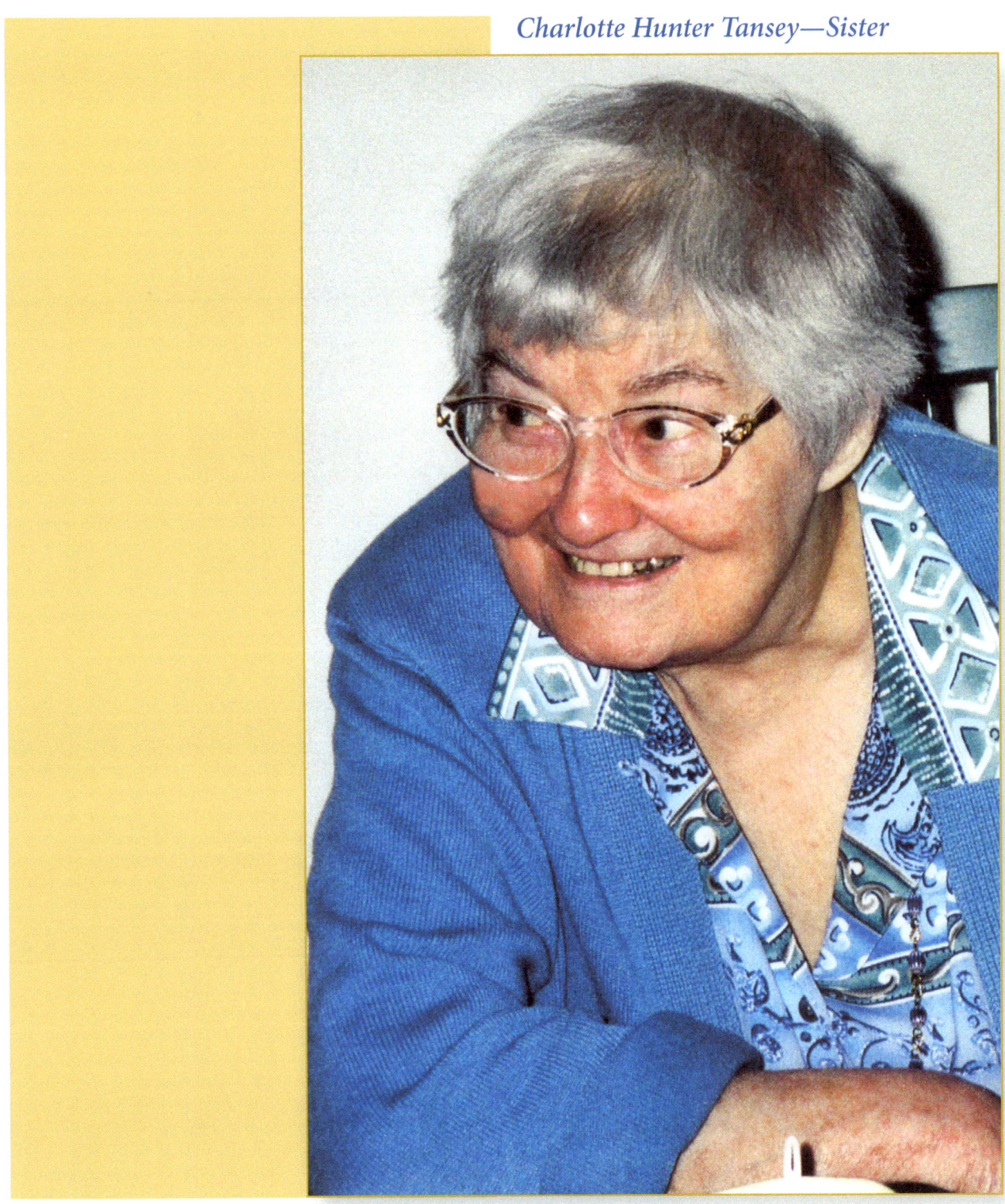

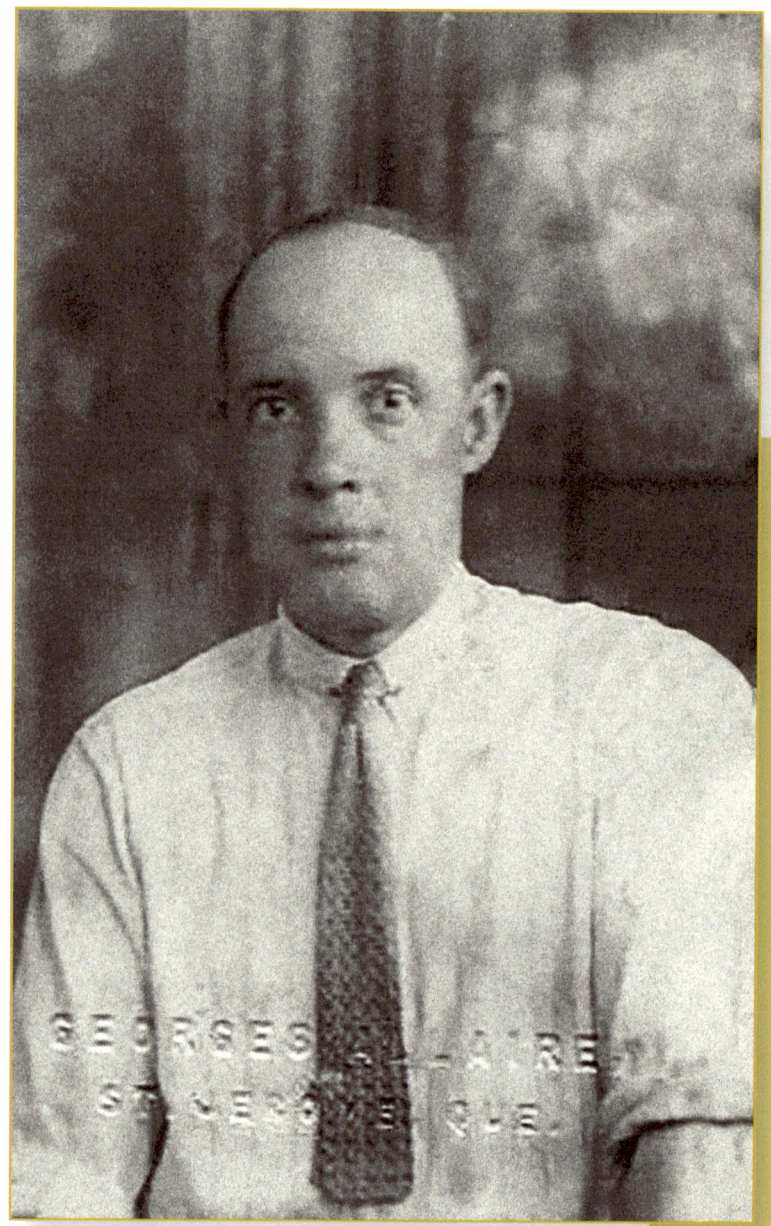

James Hunter—Uncle

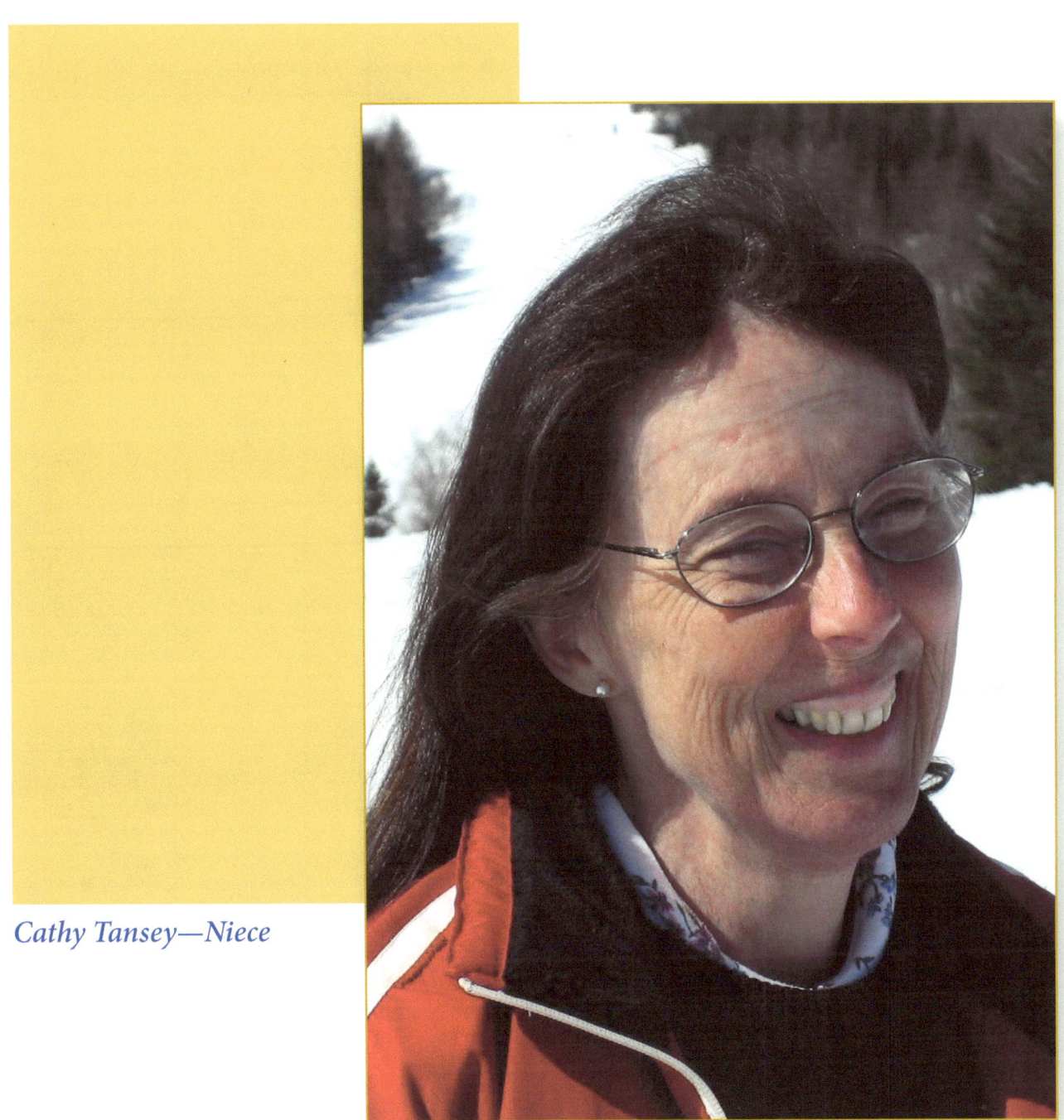

Cathy Tansey—Niece

*William Summers &
Mary (Tansey) Summers
—Sister and Brother-In-Law*
with child, Timothy Summers

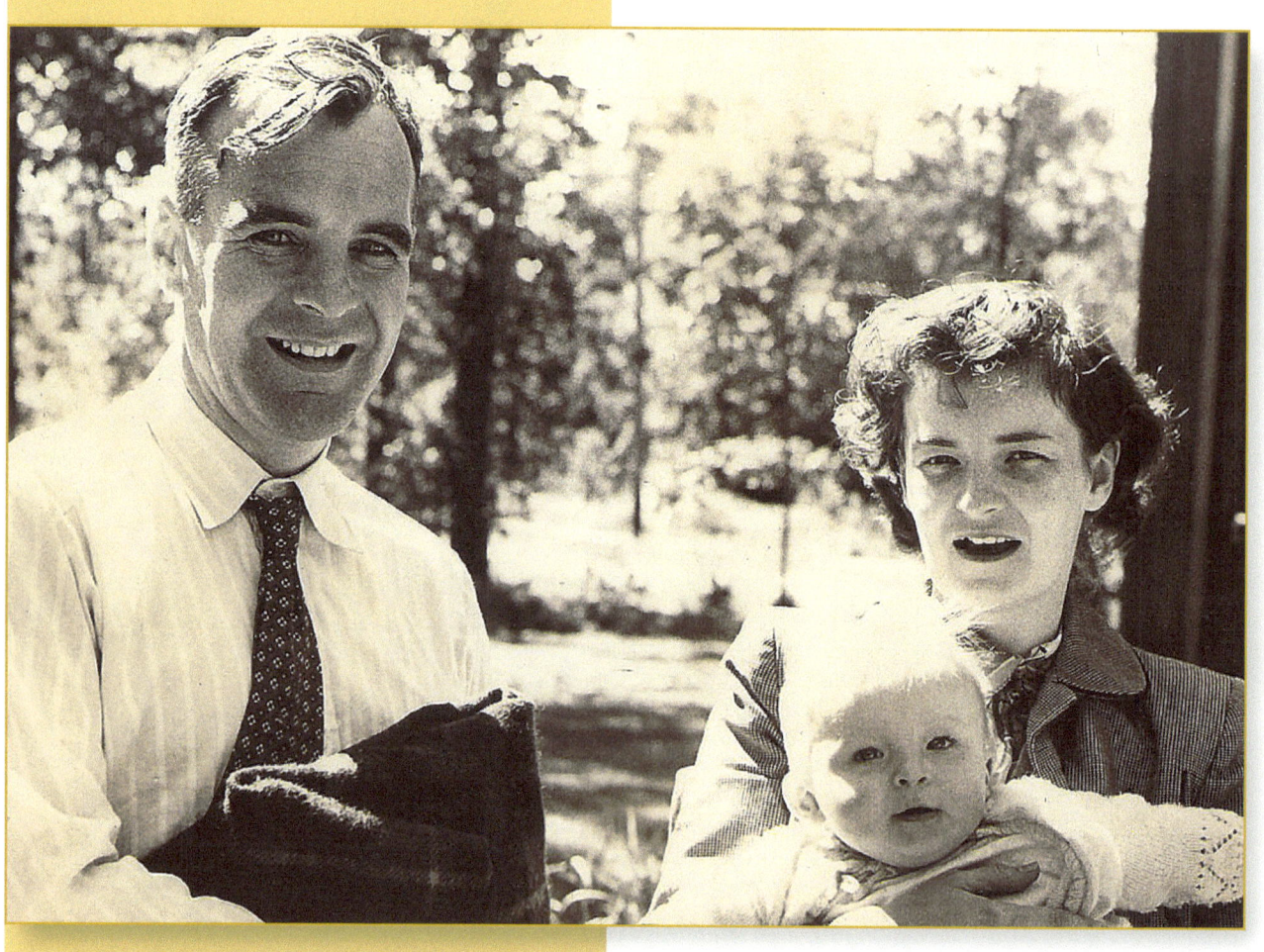

Barbara (Tansey) Cooper—Sister

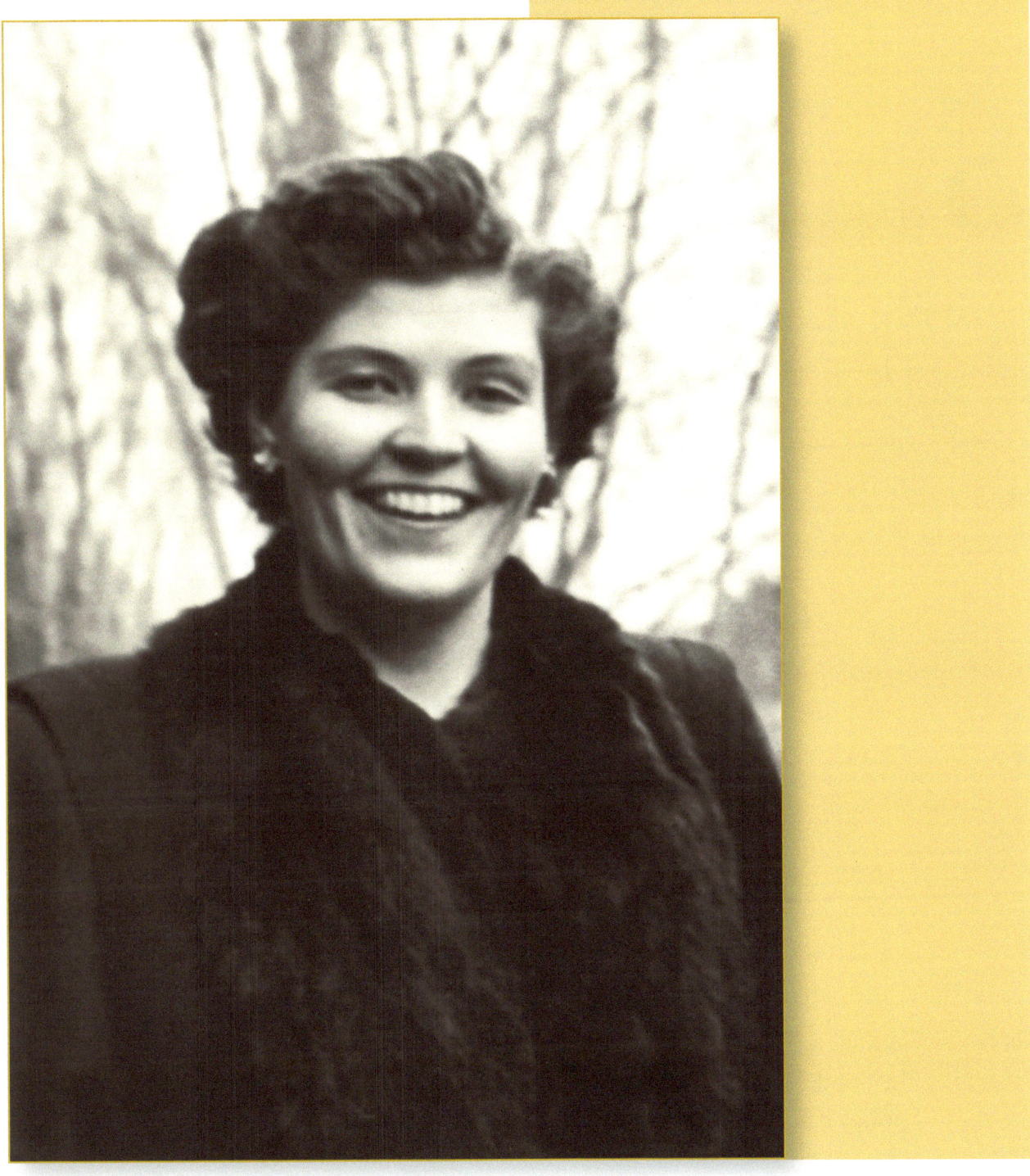

Recommendations

Since today's society has chosen to warehouse the elderly, I hope we can help to make the senior years more tolerable and even possibly more pleasant for us all.

1) Please talk to seniors as if they might just possibly have some understanding and some brains. Staff should remember that their residents, a very short time ago, had very busy and happy lives, until illness overtook them. Residents should be treated with respect, not as if every resident was an Alzheimer's Disease patient, unable to understand.

2) All staff, of the higher and lower status, should have some information about their residents. My former caregiver said she understood me better now, because her husband had had a stroke, and she understood her husband better because she had worked with me. The level of frustration was much the same for us both. With sharing some knowledge comes understanding and respect.

3) Residents should be encouraged to do as much as they are able to do, with safety, even though it may be quicker if the PAB does it instead. I am very lucky to have some caregivers who will wait a minute or two when I try to do something. It gives me such a feeling of accomplishment, instead of carrying a feeling of hopelessness.

4) Residents should have as much therapy as they can take. I would like daily therapy. Meanwhile I must understand that the budget only permits 3 times a week. I do not feel that the Government appreciates how valuable therapists are.

5) The food—I don't think anybody is happy with it. There are a few dishes that the kitchen does very nicely, so I know they are capable of more. I think the staff just needs some inspiration and a closer knowledge of the residents by some intermingling—staff

and residents. If you know a person you are more likely to think of that person's needs when preparing their dishes. Take your heaviest winter gloves, put them on and try to pick up diced carrots or tough squares of meat. That's about how difficult the task of eating those foods can be for a senior with shaky hands. Then, try cutting the meat while your plate keeps circling around on your tray.

6) The laundry service should be improved. Since we are charged to have labels put on our clothes when we come here, then management has a responsibility for returning them. So many clothes are either lost or ruined that I do not even report them gone any more.

7) The toilets should be checked. The one in my bathroom would fit a person with long arms and short legs and an unbalanced body. It is not surprising that the other woman who shares the bathroom fell off the toilet and broke her ankle.

Also the bathroom should be cut in half and a separate toilet put in each half for hygienic reasons. Currently I am using my bedroom as a bathroom. It is crude, rude and horrible. There is a reason why it is the law to have ventilation systems in the bathrooms.

8) The elevators should have responsible persons operating them at busy times—for Mass, meals, parties or functions. My sister had many bruises from the door banging on her as she tried to get in or out. I simply will not go on the elevator alone because my chair is too long. Even if the elevator is empty I cannot turn—so I either have to go in or come out backwards. The floor buttons on the elevators should be more distinct—they are very hard to see with seniors' eyes.

9) Some time ago, I asked that one wall in my room be painted as it has 3 areas where the paint is missing. It looks like the slums. I was told that the rooms would soon be painted. Nothing has happened yet! I have been in this room 5 years and not a bit of paint has come near it since or before I came in.

10) The curtains are finished in my room. They should be replaced by blinds that pull

up and down, not side to side, so that air can get in when the weather is warm.

11) My bed attacks me when I use it for support. Are we waiting until it finishes me off before it is replaced? It has been on order for about 6 months. Also the rollers move very slowly on the table. They are gummed up by hair and need regular cleaning.

12) Perhaps there should be better supervision on the nursing staff. Look at the page on Nursing Care and read again how a nurse could try to give me three pills that were not mine. Perhaps it was followed up, but not to me. Another time some cream was applied in my eyes instead of simple eye drops. I feared I was going blind.

13) One wonders if the Montreal Coroner was right in suggesting that he should ask for cause of death on Nursing Home death certificates. I wonder how many would say suicide from hopelessness, or due to negligent supervision, or careless assistance, or wrongful medication!

14) Authority figures have got to be straightforward with the public, and their residents, if they want to have any credibility.

About the Author

Carol Tansey is a Senior—83 years of age.

She was on Staff for 5 years in a Nursing Home. She has been 5 years as a Resident in a Nursing Home. She was 6 months in hospital as a patient. She was 11 months in a previous long-term care facility.

Carol studied Nutrition at Macdonald College of McGill University. In 1980, she also received a Certificate in Management in Health & Social Services, also from McGill.

She has led Discussion Groups in Seniors' Homes for 11 years. She has catered parties for as many as 200 people.

She has also written two cookbooks *(100 Gluten Free Soups & 43 Gluten Free Dinners)* which, along with this title, are available for purchase on Amazon.com. This title is also available at CreateSpace—*https://www.createspace.com/4512597*

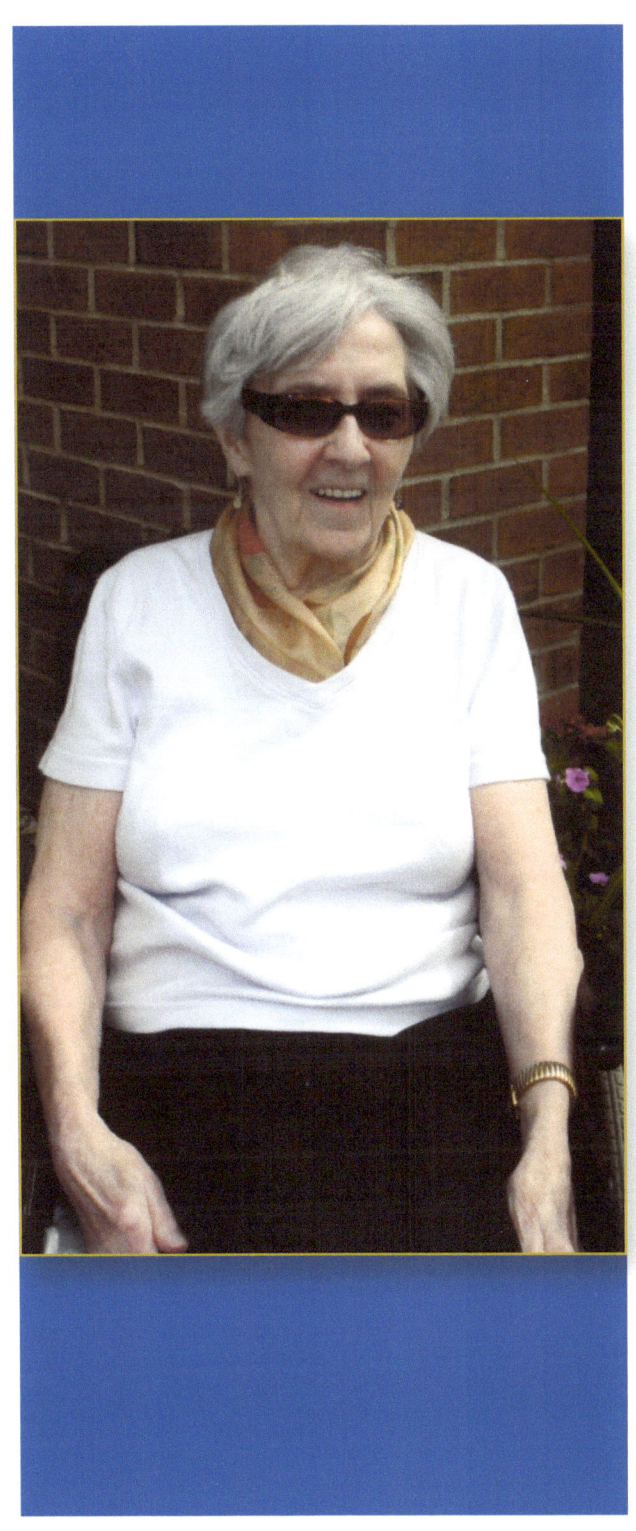

www.ingramcontent.com/pod-product-compliance
Lightning Source LLC
LaVergne TN
LVHW071025070426
835507LV00002B/35